MADE SIMPLE™
KETO

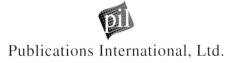

Publications International, Ltd.

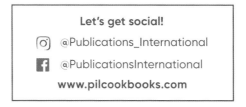

Let's get social!

@Publications_International

@PublicationsInternational

www.pilcookbooks.com

CONTENTS

THE KETOGENIC DIET AND DIETING

The ketogenic diet is hardly new. The idea that fasting could be used as a therapy to treat disease was one that ancient Greek and Indian physicians embraced. "On the Sacred Disease," an early treatise in the Hippocratic Corpus, proposed how dietary modifications could be useful in epileptic management. Hippocrates, a Greek physician called the Father of Modern Medicine, wrote in "Epidemics" how abstinence from food and drink cured epilepsy.

In the 20th century, the first ketogenic diet became popularized in the 1920's and 30's as a regimen for treating epilepsy and an alternative to non-mainstream fasting. It was also promoted as a means of restoring health. In 1921, the ketogenic diet was officially established when an endocrinologist noted that three water-soluble compounds were produced by the liver as a result of following a diet that was rich in fat and low in carbohydrates. The term "water diet" had been used prior to this time to describe a diet that was free of starch and sugar. This is because when carbohydrates are broken down by the body carbon dioxide and water are by-products. When newer, anticonvulsant therapies were established, the ketogenic diet was temporarily abandoned.

In the 1960's the ketogenic diet was revisited when it was noted that more ketones are produced by medium chain triglycerides (MCTs) per unit of energy than by normal dietary fats (mostly long-chain triglycerides) because MCTs are quickly transported to the liver to be metabolized. In research diets where about 60 percent of the calories came from MCT oil, more protein and up to about three times as many carbohydrates could be consumed in comparison to "classic" ketogenic diets. This is why MCT oil is included in some ketogenic diets today.

In the 1950's and 1960's many versions of the ketogenic diet were popularized as high-protein, low-carbohydrate and a quick method of weight loss. Also at this time, the risk factors of excess fat and protein in the diet were criticized for being detrimental to health. Outside of the medical community, the ketogenic diet was not widely recognized for its therapeutic benefits so response to it was sensational in scope.

Then in the 1980's the Glycemic Index (GI) of foods and beverages was revealed that accounted for the differences in the speed of digestion of different types of carbohydrates. This explanation became the springboard for a number of ketogenic diets that were revised from years earlier. By the late 1990's the low-carb craze became one of the most popular types of dieting. Since this time, the original ketogenic diet underwent many refinements and hybrid diets developed.

Variations of the ketogenic diet continued to surface throughout the 20th century since the premise of the ketogenic diet—higher fat and protein and low carbohydrate—was used to treat diabetes and induce weight loss among other applications.

Table 1 summarizes the ketogenic diet basics. Many clinical studies examined their effectiveness and safety and their advantages and drawbacks were identified. These are condensed in **Table 2**.

Table 1

KETOGENIC DIET BASICS

Generally, the percentages of macronutrients on a ketogenic diet are as follows:

- **Fat** 60 to 75 percent of total daily calories
- **Protein** 15 to 30 percent of total daily calories
- **Carbohydrates** 5 to 10 percent of total daily calories

Both fat and protein have high priority on a ketogenic diet, with non-starchy carbohydrates completing the remaining calories. While calories are not as important on the ketogenic diet as they are for other diets, a closer examination of the contributions of these macronutrients helps to put the amounts into perspective.

If total daily calories were about 2,000, then the percentages of macronutrients on a ketogenic diet would resemble the following amounts:

- **Fat** 60 to 75 percent of total daily calories or about 1,200 to 1,500 calories
- **Protein** 15 to 30 percent of total daily calories or about 300 to 600 calories
- **Carbohydrates** 5 to 10 percent of total daily calories or about 100 to 200 calories

In selecting foods and beverages, think protein and fat first, then non-starchy carbohydrates to complete. Until you truly have a handle on what constitutes low carbohydrates, find a carbohydrate counter to help to keep you in line.

Table 2

ADVANTAGES AND DRAWBACKS OF KETOGENIC DIETS

ADVANTAGES	DRAWBACKS
<ul><li>No calorie counting or focus on portion sizes</li><li>Initial weight loss</li><li>After initial transition, hunger subsides</li><li>Improved energy</li><li>Improved blood pressure</li><li>Improved blood fats: high-density lipoproteins, cholesterol, low-density lipoproteins, triglycerides</li><li>Reduced blood sugar, C-reactive protein (marker of inflammation), insulin, waist circumference</li><li>Significant short-term weight loss possible</li></ul>	<ul><li>Hard to sustain</li><li>Limited food choices</li><li>May lead to taste fatigue</li><li>Socialization difficult</li><li>Digestive issues (such as constipation, fatty stool, nausea)</li><li>Nutrient deficiencies (such as calcium, vitamins A, C and D, B-vitamins, fiber, magnesium, selenium)</li><li>Fiber, vitamin and mineral supplements suggested</li><li>Increased urination (bladder, kidney contraindications)</li><li>Diabetes issues</li><li>Rapid, sizeable short-term weight loss concerning; long-term weight maintenance questionable</li></ul>

FAT IN HEALTH AND DISEASE

Fats are essential to the diet and health for many purposes. Fats function as the body's thermostat. The layer of fat just beneath the skin helps to keep the body warm or causes it to perspire to cool the body.

Fat contributes to bile acids, cell membranes and steroid hormones (such as estrogen and testosterone), cushions the body from shock and helps to regulate fluid balance. Too many or too few fats in the diet may influence each of these important body functions.

One of the most important roles of fat in the body is as an energy source, especially when carbohydrates are not available from the diet or are lacking in the body. When people did manual work all day and expended the calories that they consumed, they made good use of carbohydrates and fats in their diet and within their energy stores. Today's laborsaving devices and sedentary lifestyles create less need for excess carbohydrate calories—particularly if they are refined. Even a plant-based diet may be unnecessarily high in refined carbohydrate calories.

Over the years, as humans moved from a plant-based diet toward an animal-based diet, the composition of fatty acids in the American diet switched from monounsaturated and polyunsaturated fats to more saturated fats, which are associated more with cardiovascular disease. A diet that is only filled with saturated fats may not be healthy. Incorporating avocado, fish, nuts, oils and seeds and other foods that contain monounsaturated and polyunsaturated fats into your diet may help to support a healthier proportion of fats in the body for weight maintenance and good health.

Besides cardiovascular disease, excess saturated and trans fats in the human diet are associated with certain cancers, cerebral vascular disease, diabetes, obesity and metabolic syndrome (a collection of conditions that may include abnormal cholesterol or triglyceride levels, excess body fat around the waist, high blood sugar and increased blood pressure that may increase a person's risk of diabetes, heart disease and/or stroke).

THE CHOLESTEROL CONTROVERSY

Atherosclerosis, or hardening of the arteries, is not a modern disease. Rather, the association between blood cholesterol and cardiovascular disease was recognized as far back as the 1850's.

One hundred years later in the 1950's, cholesterol and saturated fats in the diet were implicated as major risk factors for cardiovascular disease. Then in the 1980's, major US health institutions established that the process of lowering blood cholesterol (specifically LDL-cholesterol) reduces the risk of heart attacks that are caused by coronary heart disease.

Some scientists questioned this conclusion that marked the unofficial start of what's been called the "cholesterol controversy." Studies of cholesterol-lowering drugs known as statins supported the idea that reducing blood cholesterol means less mortality from heart disease. Subsequent statin studies have questioned this association. Other factors aside from dietary cholesterol have since been identified that may lead to elevated blood cholesterol, such as trans fats.

The liver manufactures cholesterol, so reducing cholesterol in the diet should help to reduce blood cholesterol, coronary heart disease and the risk of heart attack. But in some individuals, the liver produces more cholesterol than the body requires and cardiovascular disease may still develop. Accordingly, dietary cholesterol does not necessarily predict cardiovascular disease or a heart attack.

> **WHAT YOU'LL LIKELY END UP WITH IS A SATISFYING EATING PLAN WITH AMPLE PROTEIN, HEALTHY FATS AND MINIMAL CARBOHYDRATES THAT MAY HELP YOU TO FEEL FULL AND LOSE WEIGHT IN THE PROCESS.**

While dietary cholesterol may be a measure for greater cardiovascular risks, cardiovascular disease and heart attacks are also dependent upon such lifestyle and genetic factors as age, diet, exercise, gender, genetics, medication and stress. Reducing hydrogenated fats, saturated fats and trans fats; incorporating mono- and polyunsaturated fats and losing weight to help better manage blood fats are other sensible measures to take.

Longer-term weight management is also a preventative measure in cardiovascular disease. Reducing cholesterol and saturated fat in the diet while integrating foods and beverages with mono- and polyunsaturated fats and oils, dietary fiber, antioxidants and other phytonutrients may lead to a decrease in overall calorie consumption and weight loss and an improvement in overall health.

SO WHAT (AND HOW) SHOULD I EAT?

If you want to lose body fat, then the general consensus is that you need to take in fewer calories than you burn for energy. For example, if you're an average woman over 40, decreasing your caloric intake may be a reasonable starting point. If you are of shorter stature and/or very inactive, or you haven't dropped any pounds after a few weeks, you may consider lowering your daily intake of calories by 100-calorie increments until you start seeing weight loss. But don't go much below 1,000 calories without your health care provider's supervision. (And be sure to check with your health care provider before making any major changes to your diet or activity level, especially if you have any serious health problems.)

Another approach to weight loss is the ketogenic diet that does not focus on calories. Instead, the ketogenic diet focuses on the composition of calories from fats, proteins and carbohydrates. Your health care provider may help you determine if this approach to eating and dieting is appropriate for you, so ask your doctor before you begin this or any other diet program.

Table 3

ACCEPTABLE FOODS, BEVERAGES AND INGREDIENTS FOR KETOGENIC DIETS

BEVERAGES
- Broth
- Hard liquor
- Nut milks
- Unsweetened coffee, tea
- Water

EGGS
- Egg whites
- Powdered eggs
- Whole eggs

FATS AND OILS
- Butter
- Cocoa butter
- Coconut butter, cream and oil
- Ghee
- Lard
- Oils: avocado oil, macadamia nut oil, MCT oil, olive oil and cold-pressed vegetable oils (flax, safflower, soybean)
- Mayonnaise

FISH AND SEAFOOD
- Anchovies
- Fish (catfish, cod, flounder, halibut, mackerel, mahi-mahi, salmon, snapper, trout, tuna)
- Shellfish (clams, crab, lobster, mussels, oysters, scallops, squid)

FRUITS AND VEGETABLES
- Avocados
- Cruciferous vegetables (broccoli, brussels sprouts, cabbage, cauliflower, kohlrabi)
- Fermented vegetables (kimchi, sauerkraut)
- Leafy greens (bok choy, chard, endive, lettuce, kale, radicchio, spinach, watercress)
- Lemon and lime juice and peel
- Mushrooms
- Non-starchy vegetables (asparagus, bamboo shoots, celery, cucumber)
- Seaweed and kelp
- Squash (spaghetti squash, yellow squash, zucchini)
- Tomatoes (used in moderation in some keto diets)

DAIRY PRODUCTS
- Crème fraîche
- Greek yogurt
- Hard cheese (aged Cheddar, feta, Parmesan, Swiss)
- Whipping cream
- Soft cheese (Brie, blue, Colby, Monterey Jack, mozzarella)
- Sour cream
- Spreadable cheese (cream cheese, cottage cheese and mascarpone)

MEATS AND POULTRY
- Beef (ground beef, roasts, steak, stew meat)
- Goat (leg, loin, rack, saddle, shoulder)
- Lamb (leg, loin, rack, ribs, shank, shoulder)
- Organ meats (heart, kidneys, liver, tongue)
- Poultry with skin (such as chicken, duck, pheasant, quail, turkey)
- Pork (bacon and sausage without fillers, ground pork, ham, pork chops, pork loin, tenderloin)
- Tofu used in moderation in some keto diets)
- Veal (double, flank, leg, rib, shoulder, sirloin)

NON-DAIRY BEVERAGES
- Almond milk
- Cashew milk
- Coconut milk
- Soymilk (used in moderation in some keto diets)

NUTS AND SEEDS
- Nut butters (almond, macadamia)
- Seeds (chia, flax, poppy, sesame, sunflower)
- Whole nuts (almonds, Brazil nuts, macadamia, pecans, hazelnuts, pine nuts, walnuts)

PANTRY ITEMS
- Herbs (dried or fresh such as basil, cilantro, oregano, parsley, rosemary and thyme)
- Horseradish
- Hot sauce
- Mustard
- Pepper
- Pesto sauce
- Pickles
- Salad dressings (without sweeteners)
- Salt
- Spices (such as ground red pepper, chili powder, cinnamon and cumin)
- Unsweetened gelatin
- Vinegar
- Whey protein (unsweetened)
- Worcestershire sauce

Table 4

UNACCEPTABLE FOODS, BEVERAGES AND INGREDIENTS FOR KETOGENIC DIETS

- Alcohol other than hard liquor (beer, sugary alcoholic beverages, wine)
- Beans
- Breads and breadstuffs
- Cakes and pastries
- Candy
- Cereals
- Cookies
- Crackers
- Flours
- Fruit, all (fresh, dried)
- Grains (amaranth, barley, buckwheat, bulgur, corn, millet, oats, rice, rye, sorghum, sprouted grains, wheat)
- Legumes (lentils, peas)
- Margarines with trans fats
- Milk (full-fat milk is acceptable in some ketogenic diets)
- Oats and muesli
- Potatoes, all kinds (white, yellow, sweet)
- Quinoa
- Pasta
- Pizza
- Processed and refined snack foods
- Rice
- Root vegetables
- Soda
- Sports drinks
- Sugar and honey
- Syrup
- Wheat gluten
- Yams

Fats are satisfying because they take longer for the body to digest, and some are converted into ketones for energy. You don't want to skimp on proteins because protein helps maintain and build calorie-burning muscle and also keeps you satiated between meals. Choose protein sources that supply monounsaturated fats and other heart-healthy unsaturated fats; good options include fish, seafood, nuts and seeds. (Fatty fish, such as herring, mackerel, salmon and tuna contain polyunsaturated fats—especially disease-fighting omega-3 fatty acids). You'll need to replace highly processed and refined foods that are full of saturated and trans fats, sugar and refined carbohydrates with minimally processed fiber- and nutrient-rich foods that include non-starchy vegetables.

What you'll likely end up with is a satisfying eating plan with ample protein, healthy fats and minimal carbohydrates that may help you to feel full and lose weight in the process. It's also a plan that may help you to maintain weight loss over time in a modified manner.

If you've ever tried to lose weight before, you know how quickly between-meal hunger may sabotage your best efforts. When your stomach starts rumbling hours before your next meal, it's tempting to grab whatever is available. Often, that "whatever" is some unhealthy packaged snack food or beverage that is loaded with empty calories, sodium, sugars and/or unhealthy fats. Or, if you manage to ignore this hunger, you may become so ravenous at the next meal that you consume far more calories than your body actually needs.

To prevent hunger from spoiling your weight-loss efforts, eat when you are hungry and stop eating when you are full, whether a meal or snack. Try to consume meals and snacks that include a source of hunger-fighting protein and healthy fat, and count your carbs so as not to exceed the daily limit of 20 to 50 grams of non-starchy carbohydrates.

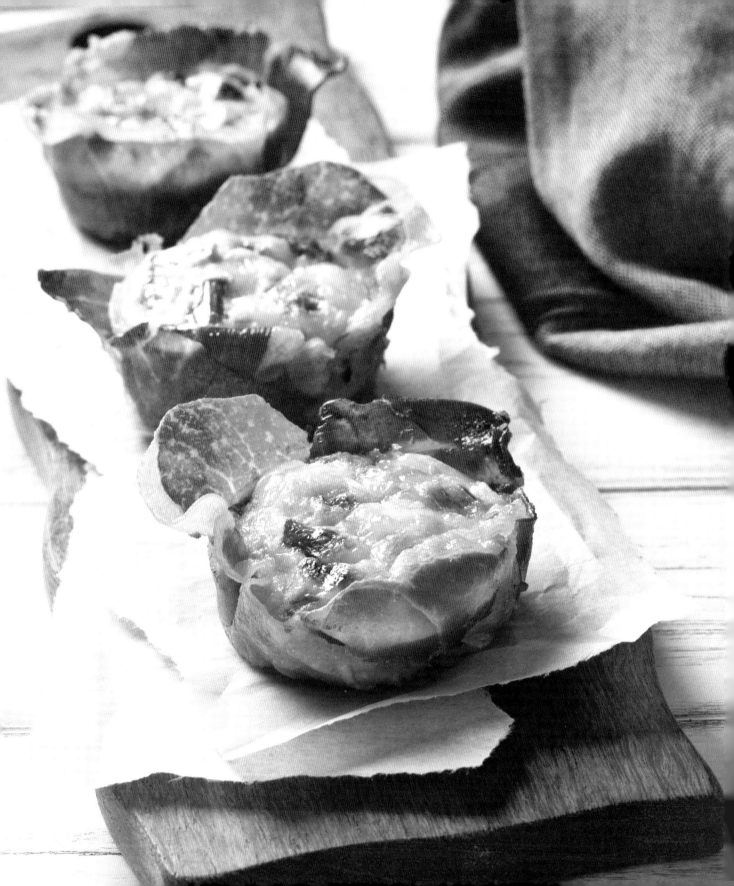

BREAKFAST

ASPARAGUS FRITTATA PROSCIUTTO CUPS
makes 6 servings

1 tablespoon olive oil

1 small red onion, finely chopped

1½ cups sliced asparagus (½-inch pieces)

1 clove garlic, minced

12 thin slices prosciutto

8 eggs

½ cup (2 ounces) grated white Cheddar cheese

¼ cup grated Parmesan cheese

2 tablespoons whipping cream

⅛ teaspoon black pepper

1 Preheat oven to 375°F. Spray 12 standard (2½-inch) muffin cups with nonstick cooking spray.

2 Heat oil in large skillet over medium heat. Add onion; cook and stir 4 minutes or until softened. Add asparagus and garlic; cook and stir 8 minutes or until asparagus is crisp-tender. Set aside to cool slightly.

3 Line each prepared muffin cup with prosciutto slice. (Prosciutto should cover cup as much as possible, with edges extending above muffin pan.) Whisk eggs, Cheddar, Parmesan, cream and pepper in large bowl until well blended. Stir in asparagus mixture. Pour into prosciutto-lined cups, filling about three-fourths full.

4 Bake about 20 minutes or until frittatas are puffed and golden brown and edges are pulling away from pan. Cool in pan 10 minutes; remove to wire rack. Serve warm or at room temperature.

PER SERVING:

calories 270, *total fat* 18g, *carbs* 5g, *net carbs* 4g, *dietary fiber* 1g, *protein* 22g

SPINACH AND HAM QUICHE

makes 4 servings

3 eggs

1 cup whole milk

¼ teaspoon salt

¼ teaspoon ground nutmeg

Pinch red pepper flakes

1 package (10 ounces) frozen chopped spinach

1 cup (4 ounces) shredded mozzarella cheese

½ cup (about 2 ounces) chopped ham

⅓ cup chopped onion

1 clove garlic, minced

Salsa (optional)

1 Preheat oven to 350°F. Spray 8-inch square baking pan with nonstick cooking spray.

2 Whisk eggs, milk, salt, nutmeg and red pepper flakes in large bowl until well blended. Stir in spinach, cheese, ham, onion and garlic; mix well. Pour into prepared pan.

3 Bake about 40 minutes or until center is firm. Serve with salsa, if desired.

PER SERVING:

calories 220, *total fat* 13g, *carbs* 8g, *net carbs* 6g, *dietary fiber* 2g, *protein* 17g

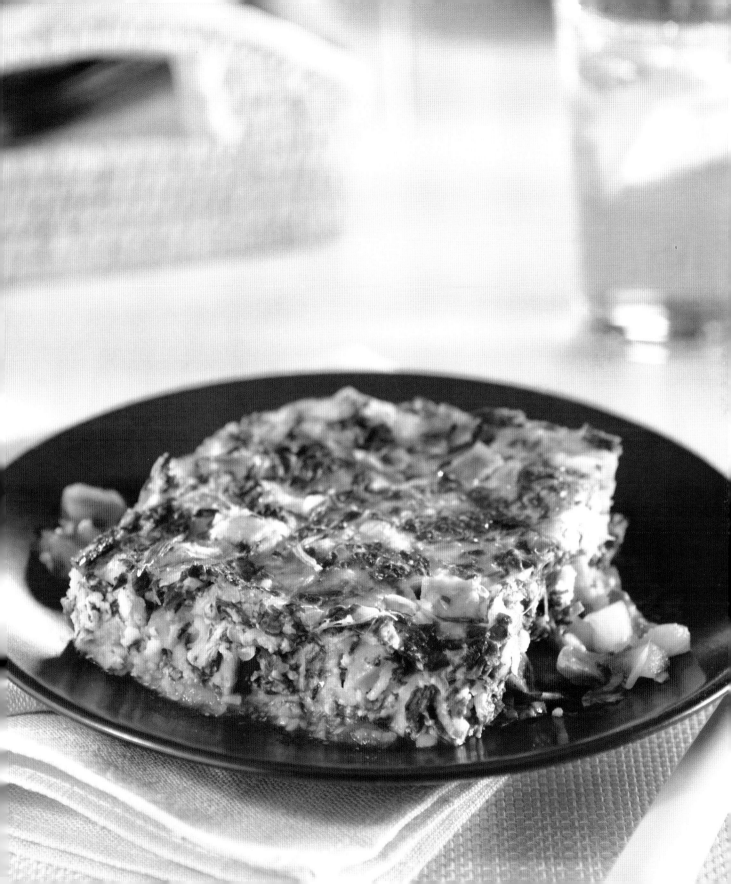

HAM AND VEGETABLE OMELET

makes 4 servings

2 ounces diced ham (about ½ cup)

1 small onion, diced

½ medium green bell pepper, diced

½ medium red bell pepper, diced

2 cloves garlic, minced

1½ cups liquid egg substitute
or 6 eggs, beaten

⅛ teaspoon black pepper

½ cup (2 ounces) shredded reduced-fat Colby cheese, divided

1 medium tomato, chopped

Hot pepper sauce (optional)

1 Spray large nonstick skillet with nonstick cooking spray; heat over medium-high heat. Add ham, onion, bell peppers and garlic; cook and stir 5 minutes or until vegetables are crisp-tender. Transfer mixture to large bowl.

2 Wipe out skillet with paper towels; spray with cooking spray. Heat over medium-high heat. Pour egg substitute into skillet; sprinkle with black pepper. Cook 2 minutes or until bottom is set, lifting edges with spatula to allow uncooked portion to flow underneath. Reduce heat to medium-low; cover and cook 4 minutes or until top is set.

3 Gently slide omelet onto large serving plate; spoon ham mixture down center. Sprinkle with ¼ cup cheese. Carefully fold two sides of omelet over ham mixture; sprinkle with remaining ¼ cup cheese and tomato. Cut into four pieces; serve immediately with hot pepper sauce, if desired.

PER SERVING:

calories 126, *total fat* 4g, *carbs* 8g, *net carbs* 7g, *dietary fiber* 1g, *protein* 16g

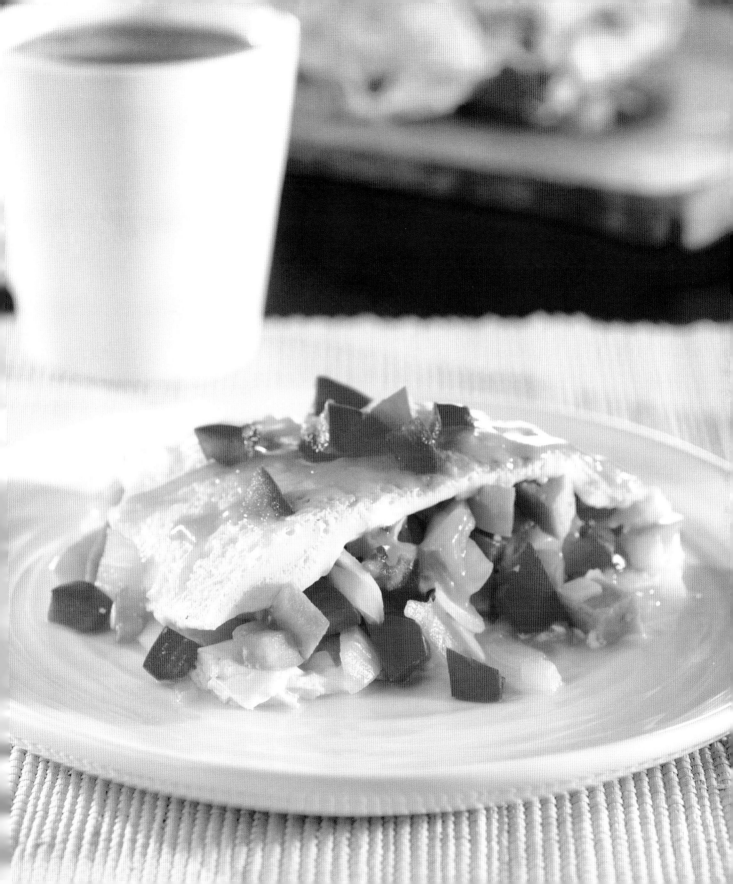

FETA BRUNCH BAKE

makes 4 servings

1 medium red bell pepper

2 packages (10 ounces each)
  fresh spinach, stemmed

6 eggs

1½ cups (6 ounces) crumbled
  feta cheese

⅓ cup chopped onion

2 tablespoons chopped fresh parsley

¼ teaspoon dried dill weed

  Dash black pepper

1 Preheat broiler. Place bell pepper on foil-lined broiler pan. Broil 4 inches from heat source 15 to 20 minutes or until blackened on all sides, turning every 5 minutes with tongs. Place in paper bag; close bag and set aside to cool 15 to 20 minutes. Remove core; cut pepper in half and rub off skin. Rinse under cold water. Cut into ½-inch pieces.* *Reduce oven temperature to 400°F.*

2 Fill medium saucepan half full of water; bring to a boil over high heat. Add spinach; return to a boil. Boil 2 to 3 minutes or until wilted. Drain spinach; immediately transfer to bowl of cold water to stop cooking. Drain and squeeze out excess water; finely chop.**

3 Spray 1-quart baking dish with nonstick cooking spray. Beat eggs in large bowl until foamy. Stir in roasted pepper, spinach, cheese, onion, parsley, dill weed and black pepper until blended. Pour into prepared dish.

4 Bake 20 minutes or until set. Let stand 5 minutes before serving.

Or use 1 jarred roasted pepper, cut into ½-inch pieces. Proceed to step 2.

**Or use 2 packages (10 ounces each) frozen chopped spinach, thawed and squeezed dry. Proceed to step 3.*

PER SERVING:

calories 280, *total fat* 18g, *carbs* 10g, *net carbs* 6g, *dietary fiber* 4g, *protein* 21g

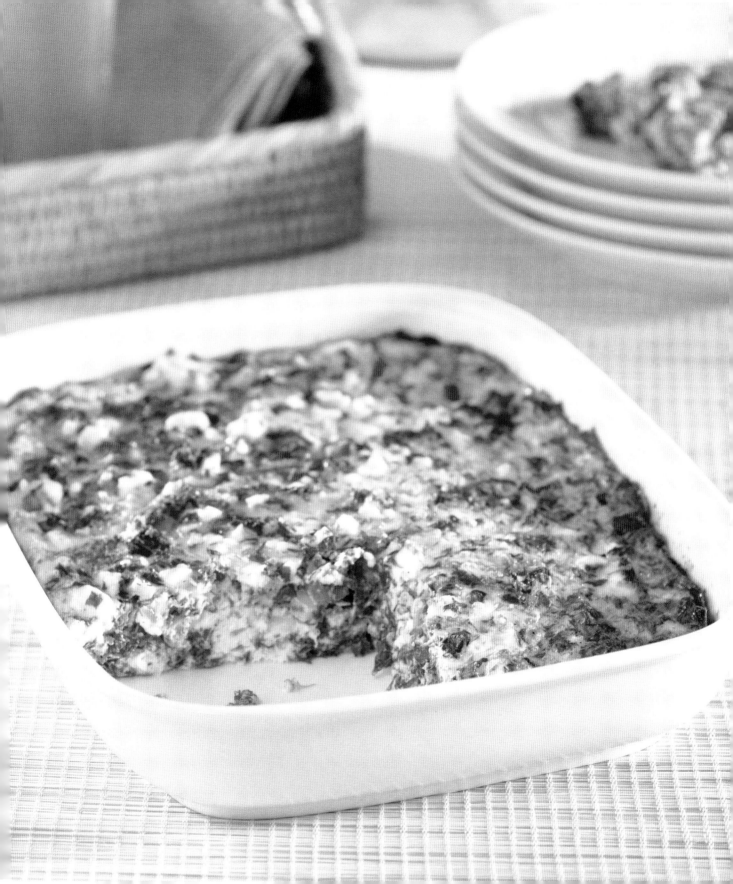

ZUCCHINI-TOMATO FRITTATA

makes 4 servings

1 cup sliced zucchini

1 cup broccoli florets

1 cup diced red or yellow bell pepper

3 whole eggs*

5 egg whites*

½ cup 1% low-fat cottage cheese

½ cup rehydrated** sun-dried tomatoes (1 ounce dry), coarsely chopped

¼ cup chopped green onions

¼ cup chopped fresh basil

⅛ teaspoon ground red pepper

2 tablespoons grated Parmesan cheese

Paprika (optional)

*Or substitute 6 whole eggs.

**To rehydrate sun-dried tomatoes, pour 1 cup boiling water over tomatoes in small bowl. Let soak 5 to 10 minutes or until softened; drain well.

1 Preheat broiler. Spray large ovenproof nonstick skillet with nonstick cooking spray; heat over medium-high heat. Add zucchini, broccoli and bell pepper; cook and stir 3 to 4 minutes or until crisp-tender.

2 Beat whole eggs, egg whites, cottage cheese, tomatoes, green onions, basil and ground red pepper in medium bowl until well blended. Pour egg mixture over vegetables in skillet. Cook 7 to 8 minutes or until frittata is almost firm and golden brown on bottom, gently lifting edges with spatula to allow uncooked portion to flow underneath. Remove from heat; sprinkle with Parmesan.

3 Broil about 5 inches from heat 3 to 5 minutes or until top is golden brown. Sprinkle with paprika, if desired. Cut into wedges; serve immediately.

PER SERVING:

calories 160, *total fat* 5g, *carbs* 13g, *net carbs* 10g, *dietary fiber* 3g, *protein* 16g

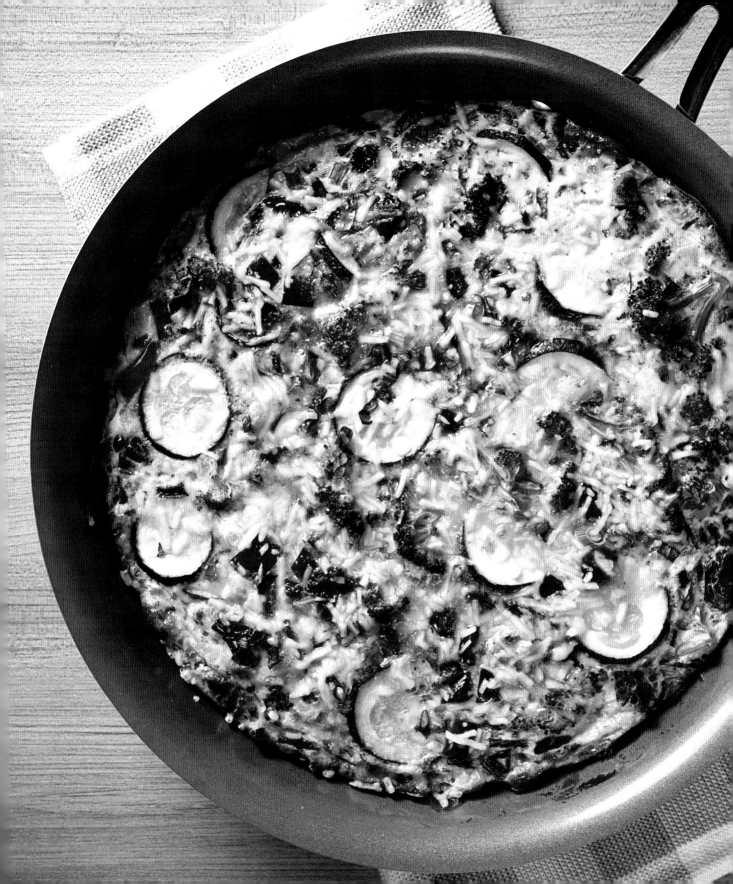

INDIVIDUAL SPINACH
AND BACON QUICHES

makes 12 servings

3 slices bacon

½ small onion, diced

1 package (10 ounces) frozen chopped spinach, thawed and squeezed dry

½ teaspoon black pepper

⅛ teaspoon ground nutmeg

Pinch salt

3 eggs, lightly beaten

1 container (15 ounces) whole-milk ricotta cheese

2 cups (8 ounces) shredded mozzarella cheese

1 cup grated Parmesan cheese

1 Preheat oven to 350°F. Spray 12 standard (2½-inch) muffin cups with nonstick cooking spray.

2 Cook bacon in large skillet over medium-high heat until crisp. Drain on paper towel-lined plate. Crumble bacon.

3 Heat skillet with bacon drippings over medium heat. Add onion; cook and stir 5 minutes or until tender. Add spinach, pepper, nutmeg and salt; cook and stir 3 minutes or until liquid is evaporated. Remove from heat; stir in bacon. Set aside to cool slightly.

4 Beat eggs in large bowl. Add ricotta, mozzarella and Parmesan; stir until well blended. Add cooled spinach mixture; mix well. Spoon evenly into prepared muffin cups.

5 Bake 40 minutes or until set. Cool in pan 10 minutes. Run thin knife around edges to loosen; remove quiches from pan. Serve warm.

PER SERVING:

calories 180, *total fat* 12g, *carbs* 4g, *net carbs* 3g, *dietary fiber* 1g, *protein* 16g

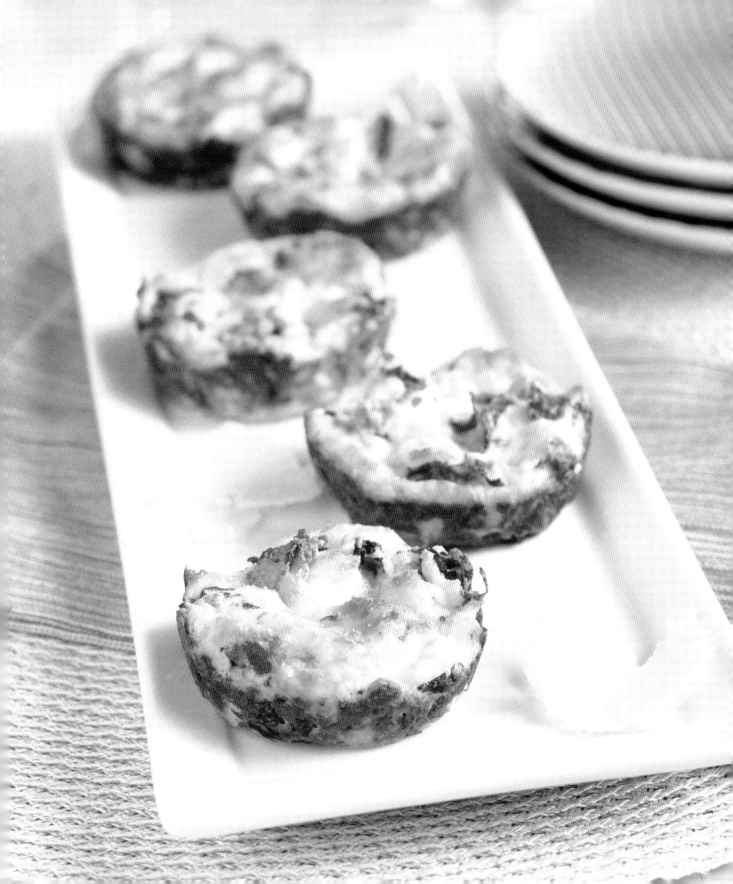

CHEDDAR SAUSAGE FRITTATA

makes 4 servings

4 eggs

¼ cup milk

1 package (12 ounces) bulk pork breakfast sausage

1 poblano pepper, seeded and chopped

1 cup (4 ounces) shredded Cheddar cheese

1 Preheat broiler. Whisk eggs and milk in medium bowl until well blended.

2 Heat large ovenproof nonstick skillet over medium-high heat. Add sausage; cook and stir 4 minutes or until no longer pink, stirring to break up meat. Remove to paper towel-lined plate. Drain off drippings.

3 Add pepper to skillet; cook and stir 2 minutes or until crisp-tender. Return sausage to skillet. Add egg mixture; stir until blended. Cover and cook over medium-low heat 10 minutes or until eggs are almost set.

4 Sprinkle cheese over frittata; broil 2 minutes or until cheese is melted. Cut into wedges; serve immediately.

PER SERVING:

calories 423, *total fat* 31g, *carbs* 4g, *net carbs* 3g, *dietary fiber* 1g, *protein* 27g

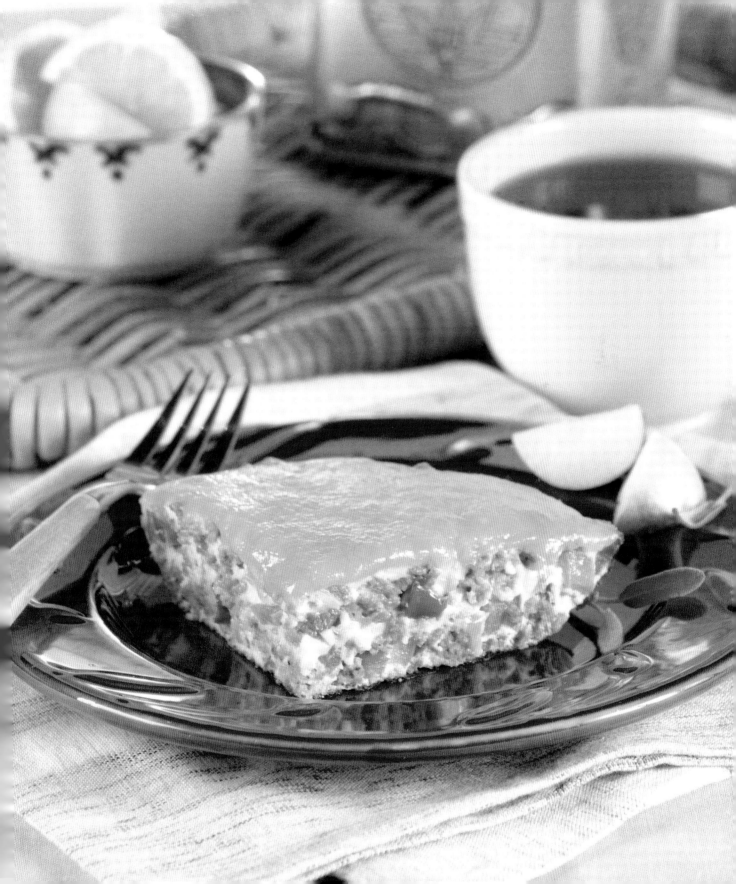

GOAT CHEESE AND TOMATO OMELET

makes 2 servings

3 egg whites

2 eggs

1 tablespoon water

⅛ teaspoon salt

⅛ teaspoon black pepper

⅓ cup crumbled goat cheese

1 medium plum tomato, diced

2 tablespoons chopped fresh basil or parsley

1 Whisk egg whites, eggs, water, salt and pepper in medium bowl until well blended.

2 Spray medium nonstick skillet with nonstick cooking spray; heat over medium heat. Add egg mixture; cook 2 minutes or until eggs begin to set on bottom, lifting edges with spatula to allow uncooked portion to flow underneath. Cook 3 minutes or until center is almost set.

3 Sprinkle cheese, tomato and basil in center of omelet. Fold half of omelet over filling; cook 1 to 2 minutes or until cheese begins to melt and center is set. Cut omelet in half; transfer to serving plates.

PER SERVING:

calories 80, *total fat* 5g, *carbs* 2g, *net carbs* 2g, *dietary fiber* 0g, *protein* 8g

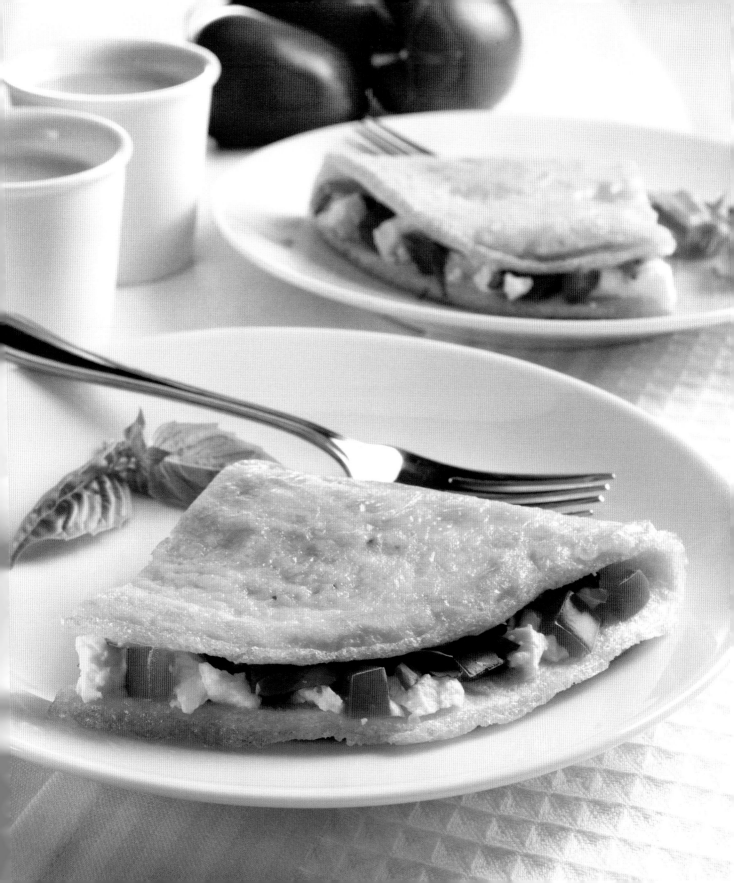

ITALIAN SAUSAGE AND ARUGULA FRITTATA

makes 4 servings

1 tablespoon olive oil

2 links sweet Italian turkey or pork sausage

2 tablespoons finely chopped red onion

12 cremini mushrooms, sliced

1 cup chopped arugula

¼ cup diced roasted red peppers

8 eggs

½ teaspoon salt

¼ teaspoon black pepper

¼ cup shredded Italian cheese blend

1 Preheat oven to 350°F. Spray four 6-ounce ramekins or custard cups with nonstick cooking spray; place on baking sheet.

2 Heat oil in medium skillet over medium heat. Remove sausage from casings; add to skillet. Cook until almost browned, stirring to break up meat. Add onion; cook and stir 1 minute or until softened. Add mushrooms; cook and stir 5 minutes. Stir in arugula and roasted peppers; cook and stir 1 minute or until heated through. Divide mixture evenly among prepared ramekins.

3 Beat eggs, salt and black pepper in medium bowl until well blended. Pour over sausage mixture; sprinkle with cheese.

4 Bake 25 to 30 minutes or until centers are set. Cool 10 minutes. (Frittatas will deflate slightly.) Serve warm or at room temperature.

PER SERVING:

calories 240, *total fat* 18g, *carbs* 4g, *net carbs* 3g, *dietary fiber* 1g, *protein* 17g

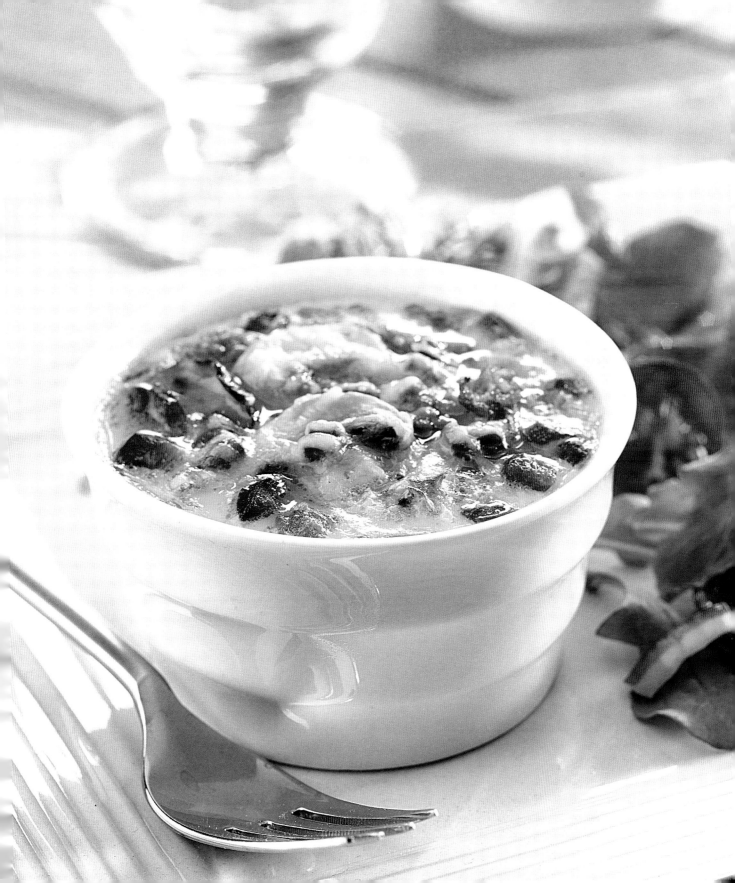

CRUSTLESS SOUTHWESTERN QUICHE

makes 4 servings

8 ounces uncooked chorizo sausage*

8 eggs

1 package (10 ounces) frozen chopped spinach, thawed and squeezed dry

1 cup crumbled queso fresco or 1 cup (4 ounces) shredded Cheddar or pepper Jack cheese

½ cup whipping cream or half-and-half

¼ cup salsa

Chorizo, a spicy Mexican pork sausage, flavored with garlic and chiles, is available in most supermarkets. If it is not available, substitute 8 ounces bulk pork sausage plus ¼ teaspoon ground red pepper.

1 Preheat oven to 400°F. Spray 10-inch quiche dish or deep-dish pie plate with nonstick cooking spray.

2 Remove sausage from casings. Crumble sausage into medium skillet; cook over medium heat until browned, stirring to break up meat. Remove from heat; drain off drippings. Cool 5 minutes.

3 Beat eggs in medium bowl. Add spinach, cheese, cream and sausage; mix well. Pour into prepared dish.

4 Bake 20 minutes or until center is set. Let stand 5 minutes before cutting into wedges. Serve with salsa.

PER SERVING:

calories 583, *total fat* 45g, *carbs* 9g, *net carbs* 7g, *dietary fiber* 2g, *protein* 36g

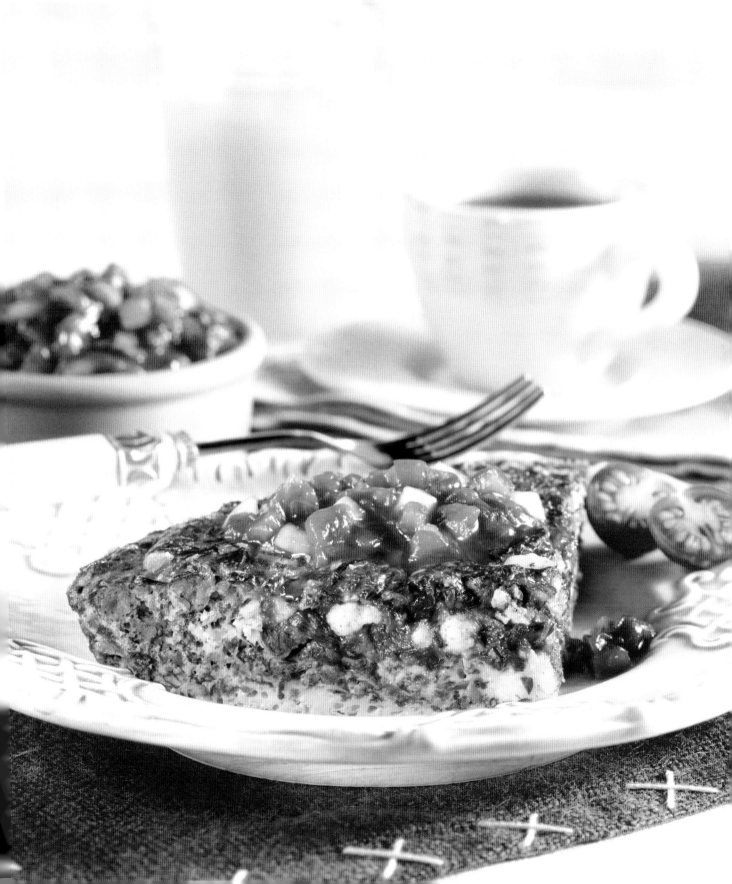

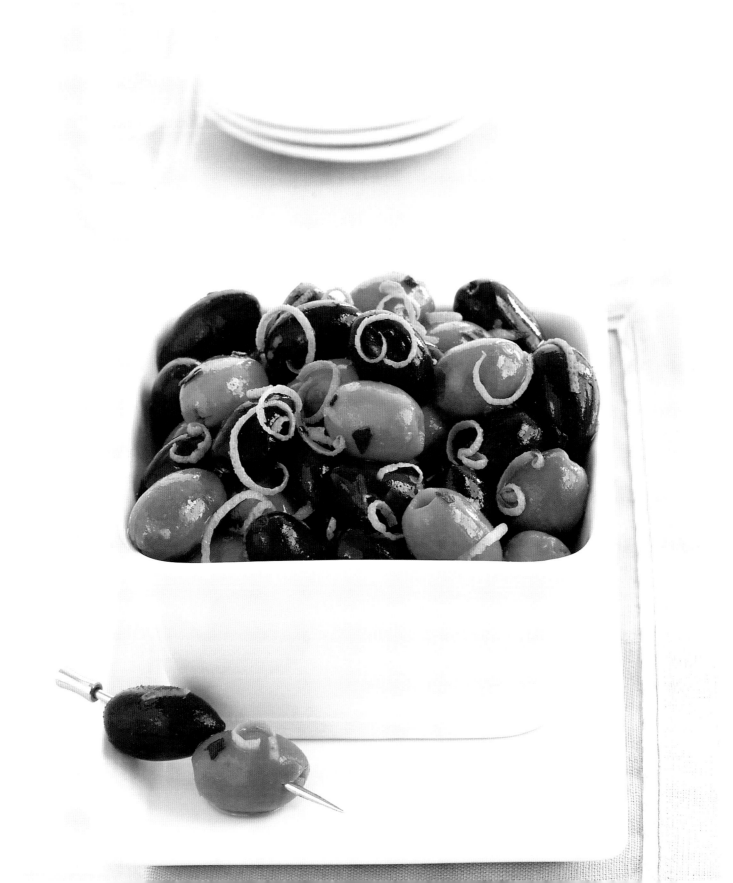

SNACKS

CITRUS-MARINATED OLIVES

makes 16 servings (2 tablespoons per serving)

1 cup (about 8 ounces) large green olives, drained

1 cup kalamata olives, rinsed and drained

⅓ cup extra virgin olive oil

¼ cup orange juice

3 tablespoons sherry vinegar or red wine vinegar

2 tablespoons lemon juice

1 tablespoon grated orange peel

1 tablespoon grated lemon peel

½ teaspoon ground cumin

¼ teaspoon red pepper flakes

Combine all ingredients in medium bowl; toss to coat. Cover and let stand overnight at room temperature; refrigerate up to 2 weeks.

PER SERVING:

calories 27, *total fat* 3g, *carbs* 1g, *net carbs* 0g, *dietary fiber* 1g, *protein* 0g

FAST GUACAMOLE AND "CHIPS"

makes 8 servings

2 ripe avocados
½ cup chunky salsa
¼ teaspoon hot pepper sauce

½ seedless cucumber, cut into ⅛-inch-thick slices

1 Cut avocados in half; remove and discard pits. Scoop flesh into medium bowl; mash with fork.

2 Add salsa and hot pepper sauce; mix well. Transfer guacamole to serving bowl; serve with cucumber "chips."

PER SERVING:

calories 85, *total fat* 7g, *carbs* 5g, *net carbs* 3g, *dietary fiber* 2g, *protein* 2g

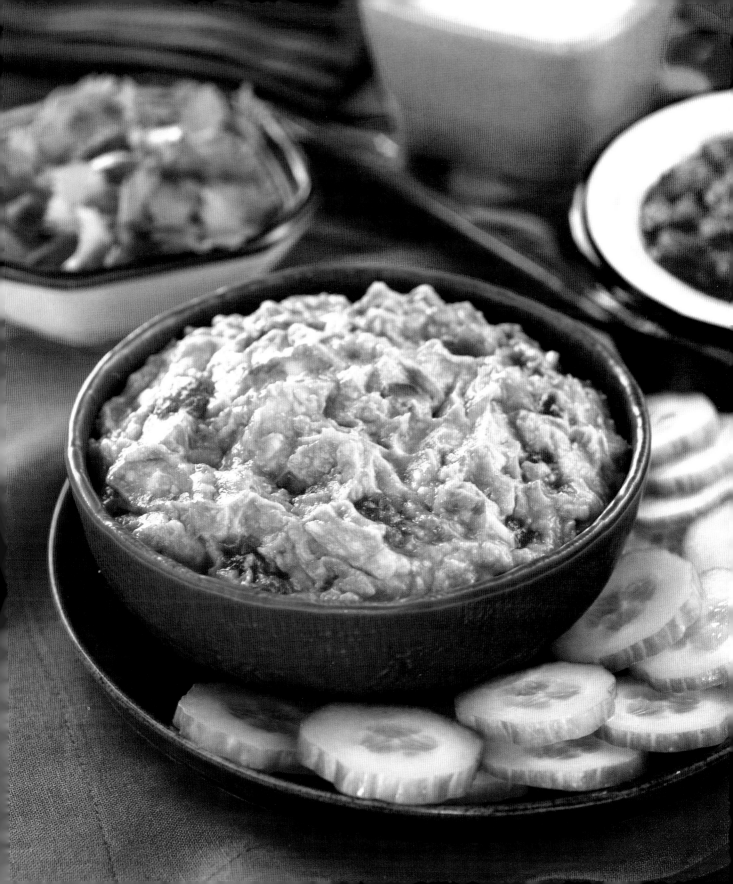

SPICY DEVILED EGGS

makes 6 servings

6 eggs
3 tablespoons whipping cream
1 green onion, finely chopped
1 tablespoon white wine vinegar
2 teaspoons Dijon mustard

½ teaspoon curry powder
½ teaspoon hot pepper sauce
3 tablespoons bacon, crisp-cooked and crumbled
1 tablespoon chopped fresh chives (optional)

1 Bring medium saucepan of water to a boil over medium-high heat. Carefully add eggs; reduce heat to maintain a gentle boil. Cook 12 minutes. Drain and rinse under cold water to stop cooking. Peel eggs; cool completely.

2 Cut eggs in half lengthwise. Place yolks in medium bowl; mash with fork. Stir in cream, green onion, vinegar, mustard, curry powder and hot pepper sauce until blended.

3 Spoon or pipe egg yolk mixture into centers of egg whites. Arrange eggs on serving plate; sprinkle with bacon. Garnish with chives.

PER SERVING:
calories 89, *total fat* 6g, *carbs* 1g, *net carbs* 0g, *dietary fiber* 1g, *protein* 6g

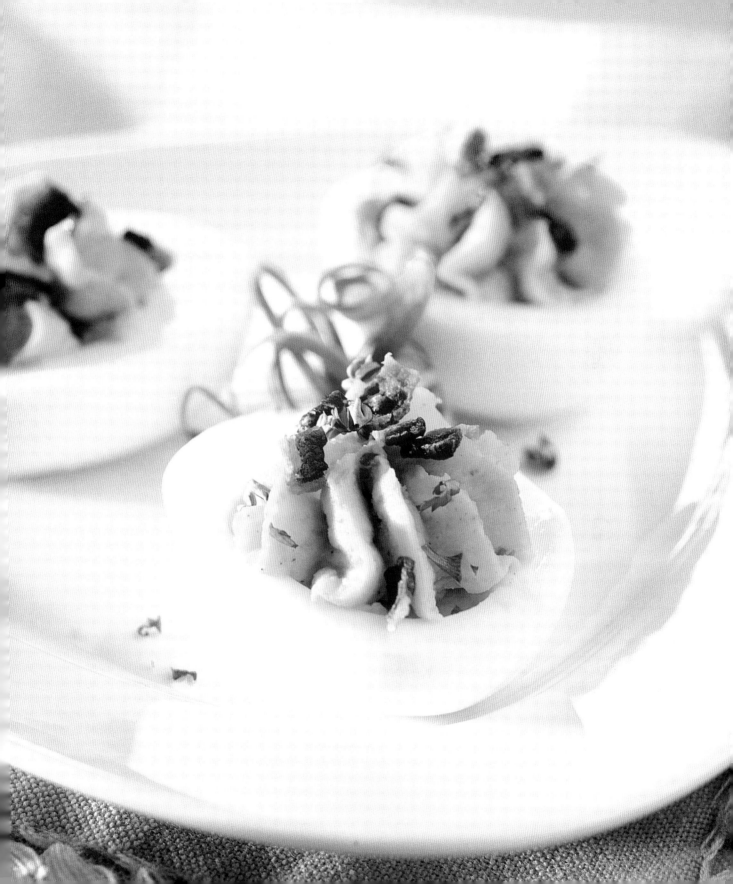

ASPARAGUS AND HAM BUNDLES

makes 6 servings

12 asparagus spears	6 large eggs
1 tablespoon olive oil	6 slices boiled ham
Salt and black pepper	
6 green onions, white parts chopped and green tops reserved	

1 Preheat oven to 350°F. Place asparagus on baking sheet. Drizzle with oil; sprinkle with salt and pepper. Roast about 10 minutes or until crisp-tender. Remove from oven; keep warm.

2 Meanwhile, heat small nonstick skillet over medium heat. Add 1 tablespoon chopped green onion; cook and stir 30 seconds. Beat 1 egg in small bowl; add to skillet, tilting skillet to spread egg in circle. *Do not stir.* Place ham slice on top of egg crêpe; cook until egg is set. Remove from pan. Repeat with remaining green onions, eggs and ham.

3 Place 2 asparagus spears on each egg crêpe; roll up. Tie bundles with reserved green onion tops, if desired. Serve immediately.

VARIATION: Top ham with shredded Swiss cheese.

PER SERVING:

calories 124, *total fat* 8g, *carbs* 2g, *net carbs* 1g, *dietary fiber* 1g, *protein* 11g

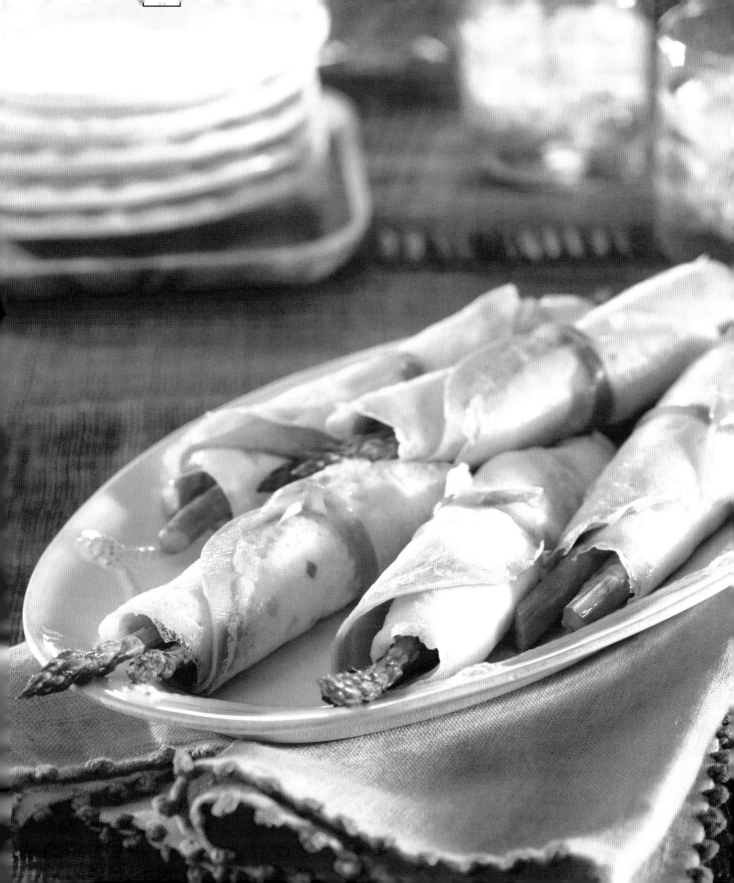

BAGNA CAUDA

makes 10 to 12 servings

¾ **cup olive oil**

6 **tablespoons butter, softened**

12 **anchovy fillets, drained**

6 **cloves garlic, peeled**

⅛ **teaspoon red pepper flakes**

Fresh vegetables for dipping:
endive spears, cauliflower florets, cucumber spears, zucchini spears, red bell pepper strips and/or sugar snap peas

SLOW COOKER DIRECTIONS

1 Combine oil, butter, anchovies, garlic and red pepper flakes in food processor; process until smooth. Transfer to small slow cooker.

2 Cover; cook on LOW 2 hours or on HIGH 1 hour or until mixture is heated through. *Turn slow cooker to LOW or WARM.* Serve with assorted dippers.

TIP: Bagna cauda is a warm Italian dip similar to fondue. The name means "warm bath" in Italian.

PER SERVING:
calories 220, *total fat* 24g, *carbs* 1g, *net carbs* 1g, *dietary fiber* 0g, *protein* 2g

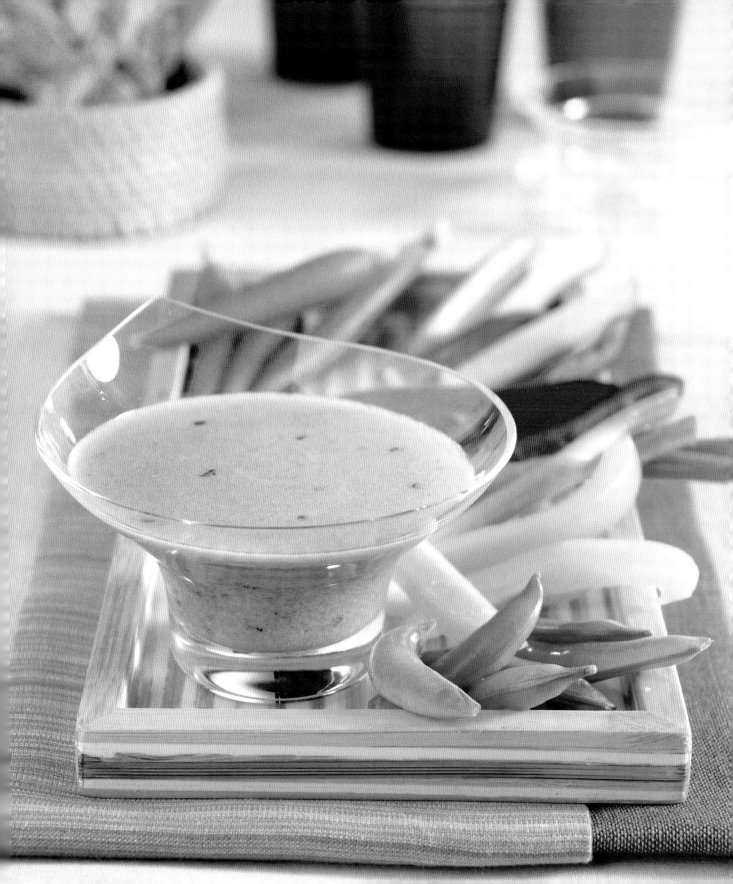

CRISPY CHEESE CHIPS

makes 8 servings

1½ cups (6 ounces) shredded mozzarella cheese*

½ cup grated Parmesan cheese

4 green onions

1 teaspoon chili powder

1 teaspoon black pepper

*Shred cheese using largest holes on box grater.

1 Place mozzarella into colander with large holes; shake to separate large shreds of cheese from smaller shreds. Save smaller shreds for another use. Transfer large shreds of cheese to medium bowl; add Parmesan and toss to blend.

2 Cut single slit in each green onion by running tip of paring knife down length of each green top once. Slice green tips crosswise into thin ribbons and add to bowl with cheese. Add chili powder and pepper; stir gently until blended.

3 Spray medium nonstick skillet with nonstick cooking spray; heat over medium-high heat. Sprinkle about ½ to 1 tablespoon cheese mixture in single layer in skillet making lacy 2-inch circle. Cook 1 to 1½ minutes until cheese melts and turns golden brown. Immediately remove from skillet with thin spatula; cool completely on parchment-lined baking sheet. Repeat with remaining cheese mixture. Store in airtight container until ready to serve.

NOTE: Cheese crisps are extremely hot and pliable when they are first removed from the skillet but they become crispy and chewy as they cool. They are easily molded if draped over a rolling pin instead of being cooled on a baking sheet.

PER SERVING:

calories 88, *total fat* 6g, *carbs* 2g, *net carbs* 2g, *dietary fiber* 0g, *protein* 7g

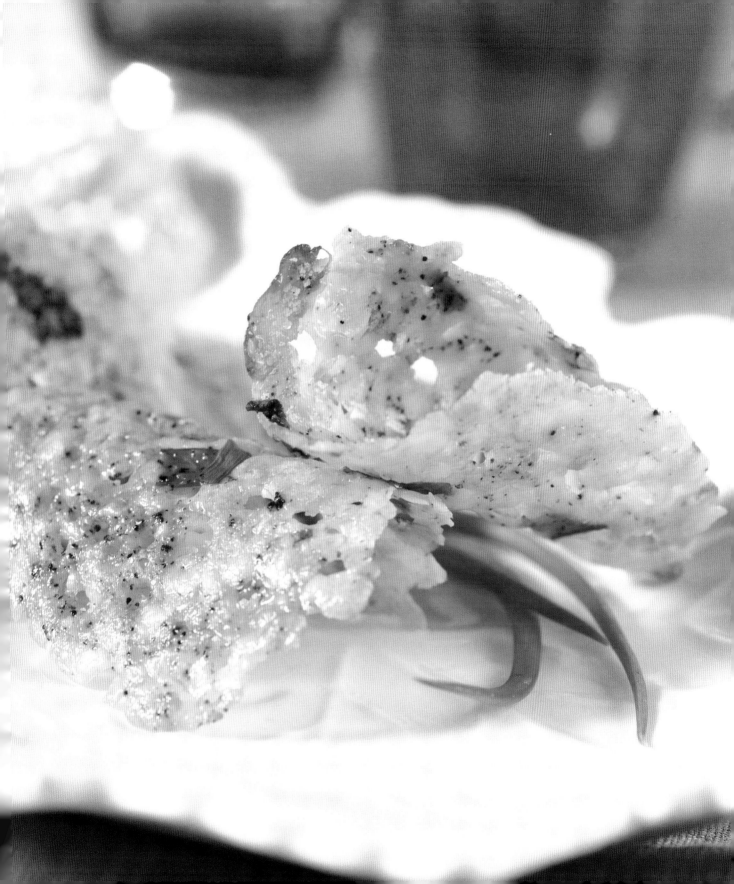

ROSEMARY NUT MIX

makes 32 servings

2 tablespoons butter

2 cups pecan halves

1 cup unsalted macadamia nuts

1 cup walnuts

1 teaspoon dried rosemary

½ teaspoon salt

¼ teaspoon red pepper flakes

1 Preheat oven to 300°F.

2 Melt butter in large saucepan over low heat. Add pecans, macadamia nuts and walnuts; stir to coat. Add rosemary, salt and red pepper flakes; cook and stir about 1 minute. Spread mixture on ungreased baking sheet.

3 Bake 8 to 10 minutes, stirring occasionally. Cool completely on baking sheet on wire rack.

PER SERVING:

calories 108, *total fat* 11g, *carbs* 2g, *net carbs* 1g, *dietary fiber* 1g, *protein* 2g

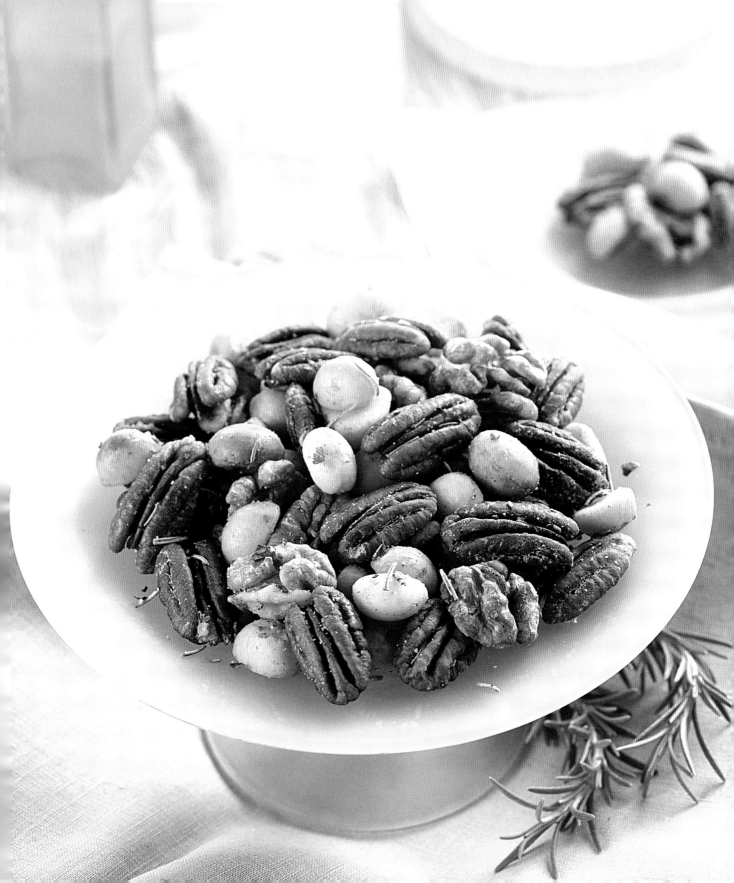

KALE CHIPS

makes 6 servings

1 large bunch kale (about 1 pound)
1 to 2 tablespoons olive oil

1 teaspoon garlic salt or other seasoned salt

1 Preheat oven to 350°F. Line baking sheets with parchment paper.

2 Wash kale and pat dry with paper towels. Remove and discard center ribs and stems. Cut leaves into 2- to 3-inch-wide pieces.

3 Combine kale leaves, oil and garlic salt in large bowl; toss to coat. Spread in single layer on prepared baking sheets.

4 Bake 10 to 15 minutes or until edges are lightly browned and leaves are crisp.* Cool completely on baking sheets. Store in airtight container.

If the leaves are lightly browned but not crisp, turn oven off and let chips stand in oven until crisp, about 10 minutes. Do not keep oven on as chips will burn easily.

PER SERVING:

calories 60, *total fat* 3g, *carbs* 7g, *net carbs* 4g, *dietary fiber* 3g, *protein* 3g

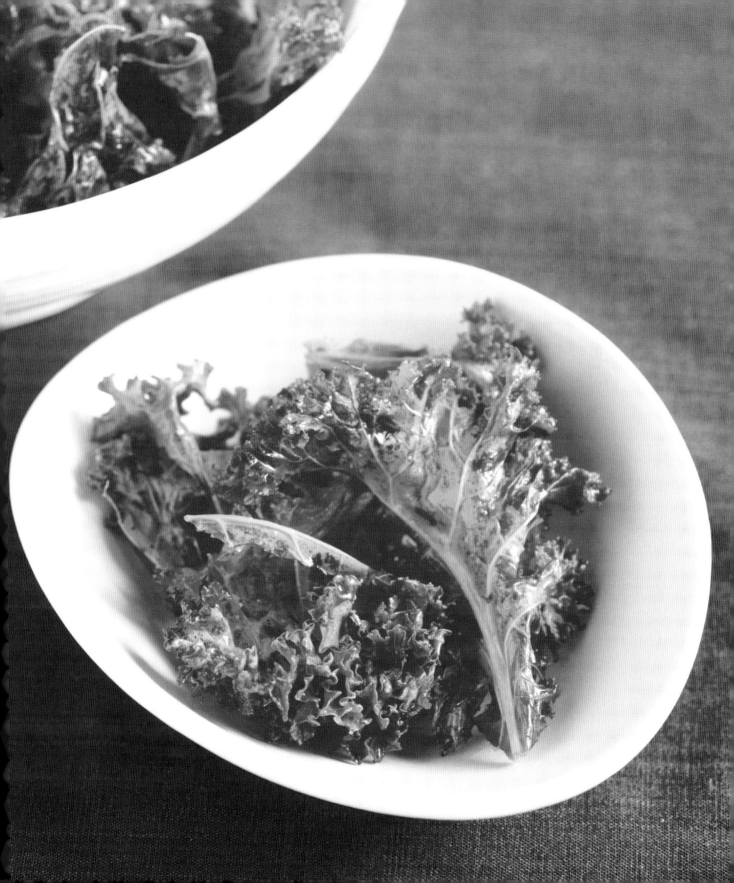

AVOCADO SALSA

makes 16 servings

1 medium avocado, diced

1 cup chopped onion

1 cup chopped seeded peeled cucumber

1 Anaheim pepper,* seeded and chopped

½ cup chopped fresh tomato

2 tablespoons chopped fresh cilantro, plus additional for garnish

½ teaspoon salt

¼ teaspoon hot pepper sauce

*Anaheim peppers can sting and irritate the skin, so wear rubber gloves when handling peppers and do not touch your eyes.

1 Combine avocado, onion, cucumber, Anaheim pepper, tomato, 2 tablespoons cilantro, salt and hot pepper sauce in medium bowl; mix gently. Cover and refrigerate at least 1 hour before serving.

2 Transfer salsa to serving bowl; garnish with additional cilantro.

PER SERVING:

calories 26, *total fat* 2g, *carbs* 2g, *net carbs* 0g, *dietary fiber* 2g, *protein* 2g

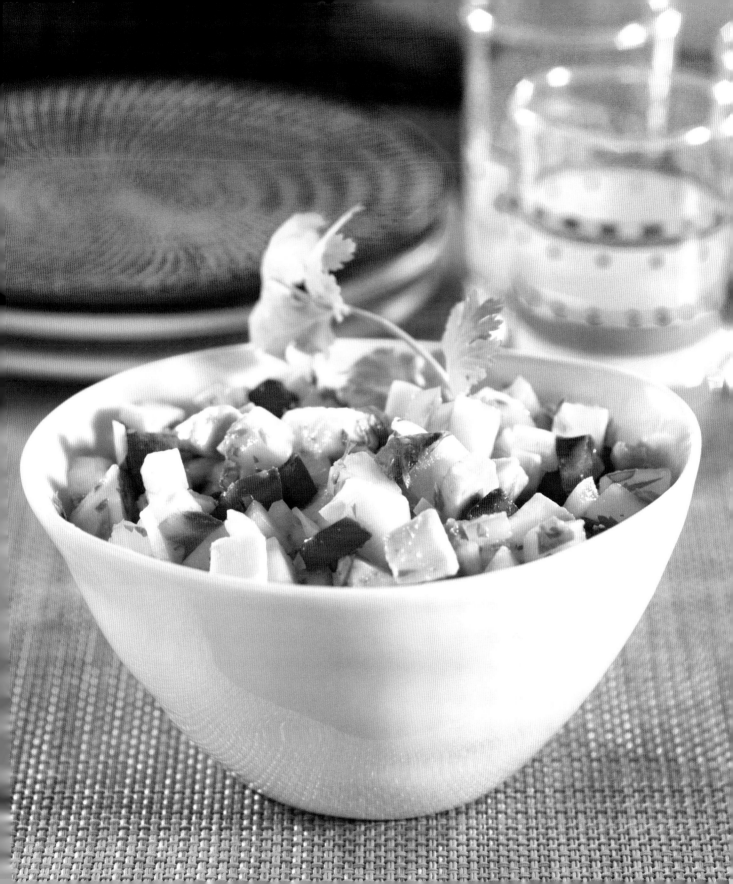

KETO BREAD

makes 1 loaf (16 servings)

7 tablespoons butter, divided

2 cups almond flour

3½ teaspoons baking powder

½ teaspoon salt

6 eggs at room temperature, separated*

¼ teaspoon cream of tartar

*Discard 1 egg yolk.

1 Preheat oven to 375°F. Generously grease 8×4-inch loaf pan with 1 tablespoon butter. Melt remaining 6 tablespoons butter in small bowl; cool slightly.

2 Combine almond flour, baking powder and salt in medium bowl. Add melted butter and 5 egg yolks; stir until blended.

3 Combine egg whites and cream of tartar in medium bowl of electric stand mixer; attach whip attachment to mixer. Whip egg whites at high speed 1 to 2 minutes or until stiff peaks form.

4 Stir one third of egg whites into almond flour mixture until well blended. Gently fold in remaining egg whites until completely blended. Scrape batter into prepared pan; smooth top.

5 Bake 25 to 30 minutes or until top is golden brown and dry and toothpick inserted into center comes out clean. Cool in pan 10 minutes; remove to wire rack to cool completely.

PER SERVING:

calories 156, *total fat* 13g, *carbs* 4g, *net carbs* 2g, *dietary fiber* 2g, *protein* 5g

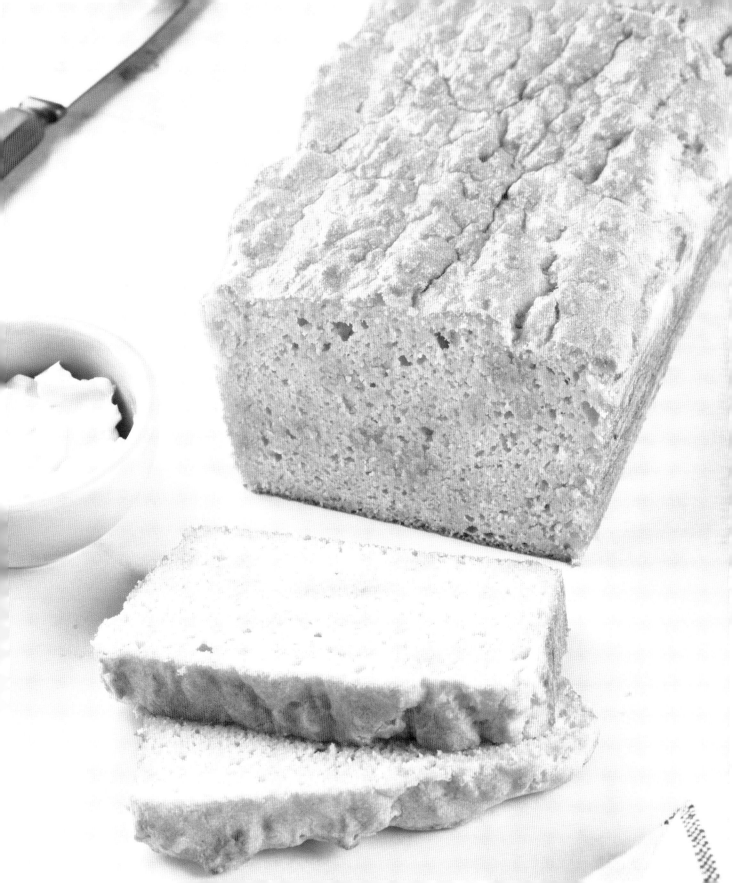

SMOKED SALMON OMELET ROLL-UPS

makes 6 servings (4 pieces per serving)

4 **eggs**

⅛ **teaspoon black pepper**

¼ **cup chive and onion cream cheese, softened**

1 **package (about 4 ounces) smoked salmon, cut into bite-size pieces**

1 Beat eggs and pepper in small bowl until well blended (no streaks of white showing). Spray large nonstick skillet with nonstick cooking spray; heat over medium-high heat.

2 Pour half of egg mixture into skillet; tilt skillet to completely coat bottom with thin layer of eggs. Cook without stirring 2 to 4 minutes or until eggs are set. Use thin spatula to carefully loosen omelet from skillet; slide onto cutting board. Repeat with remaining egg mixture to make second omelet.

3 Spread 2 tablespoons cream cheese over each omelet; top with smoked salmon. Roll up omelets tightly; wrap with plastic wrap and refrigerate at least 30 minutes.

4 Cut off ends of omelet rolls; cut crosswise into ½-inch slices.

PER SERVING:

calories 100, *total fat* 5g, *carbs* 1g, *net carbs* 1g, *dietary fiber* 0g, *protein* 14g

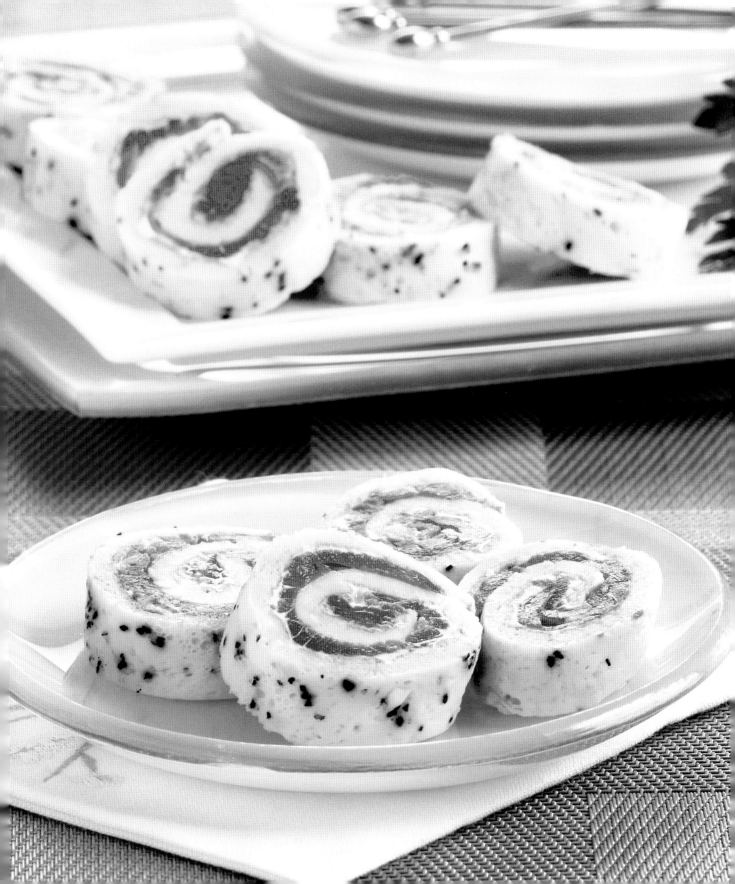

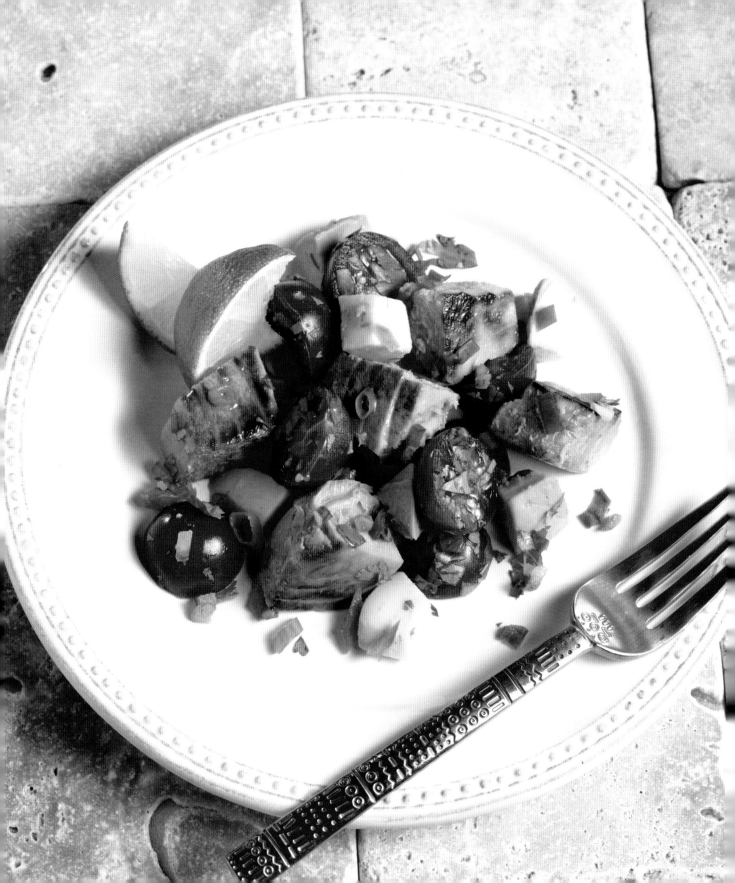

SALADS

SOUTHWESTERN TUNA SALAD

makes 4 servings

2 limes, juiced, divided

12 ounces raw tuna steaks (about 1 inch thick)

1 pint cherry or grape tomatoes, halved

¼ cup diced ripe avocado

1 jalapeño pepper,* seeded and minced

1 green onion, chopped (green part only)

1 tablespoon chopped fresh cilantro

1½ teaspoons avocado oil

¼ teaspoon salt

¼ teaspoon ground cumin

⅛ teaspoon black pepper

Lime wedges (optional)

*Jalapeño peppers can sting and irritate the skin, so wear rubber gloves when handling peppers and do not touch your eyes.

1 Place juice of one lime in glass baking dish or shallow bowl. Add tuna; turn to coat. Marinate at room temperature 30 minutes, turning once.

2 Spray stovetop grill pan with nonstick cooking spray; heat over medium heat 30 seconds. Add tuna; cook 5 to 6 minutes per side. Remove to plate; cool to room temperature. Cut into bite-size chunks.

3 Combine tuna, tomatoes, avocado, jalapeño, green onion and cilantro in large bowl.

4 Whisk oil, remaining lime juice, salt, cumin and black pepper in small bowl until well blended. Pour over salad; toss gently to coat. Serve with lime wedges, if desired.

PER SERVING:

calories 180, *total fat* 7g, *carbs* 8g, *net carbs* 5g, *dietary fiber* 3g, *protein* 21g

ANTIPASTO SALAD

makes about 5 cups (12 appetizer servings)

¼ cup extra virgin olive oil

2 tablespoons balsamic vinegar

1 clove garlic, minced

½ teaspoon salt

¼ teaspoon black pepper

2 cups cherry tomatoes

1 can (about 14 ounces) quartered
artichoke hearts, drained

8 ounces small balls or cubes
fresh mozzarella cheese

1 cup drained pitted kalamata olives

¼ cup sliced fresh basil leaves

Lettuce leaves

1 Whisk oil, vinegar, garlic, salt and pepper in medium bowl until well blended. Add tomatoes, artichokes, cheese, olives and basil; toss to coat. Let stand at room temperature 30 minutes.

2 Line platter with lettuce. Arrange antipasto over lettuce; serve at room temperature.

SERVING SUGGESTION: Serve antipasto with toothpicks as an appetizer or spoon over Bibb lettuce leaves for a first-course salad.

PER SERVING:

calories 130, *total fat* 11g, *carbs* 6g, *net carbs* 3g, *dietary fiber* 3g, *protein* 5g

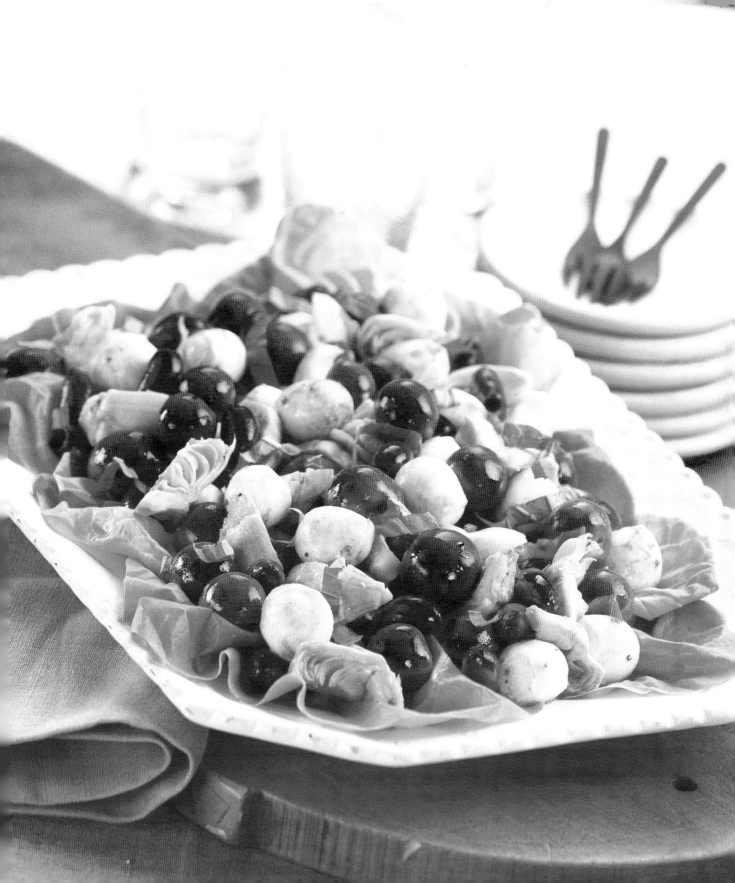

SHRIMP RÉMOULADE SALAD

makes 4 servings

12 ounces cooked shrimp, peeled and deveined (with tails on)

2 cups shredded red cabbage

2 stalks celery, finely sliced

½ cup sliced green onions

3 tablespoons ketchup

2 tablespoons prepared horseradish

1½ tablespoons white wine vinegar

1 tablespoon olive oil

1 tablespoon Dijon mustard

2 cloves garlic, minced

¼ teaspoon salt

1 package (10 ounces) frozen mustard greens or frozen spinach

1 Combine shrimp, cabbage, celery, green onions in large bowl. Whisk ketchup, horseradish, vinegar, oil, mustard, garlic and salt in small bowl until well blended. Pour over shrimp mixture; toss gently to coat. Cover and refrigerate at least 15 minutes or up to 2 days.

2 Cook mustard greens according to package directions. Cool, drain and squeeze excess water from greens. Divide greens among serving bowls or plates, top with shrimp salad.

PER SERVING:

calories 177, *total fat* 5g, *carbs* 10g, *net carbs* 6g, *dietary fiber* 4g, *protein* 21g

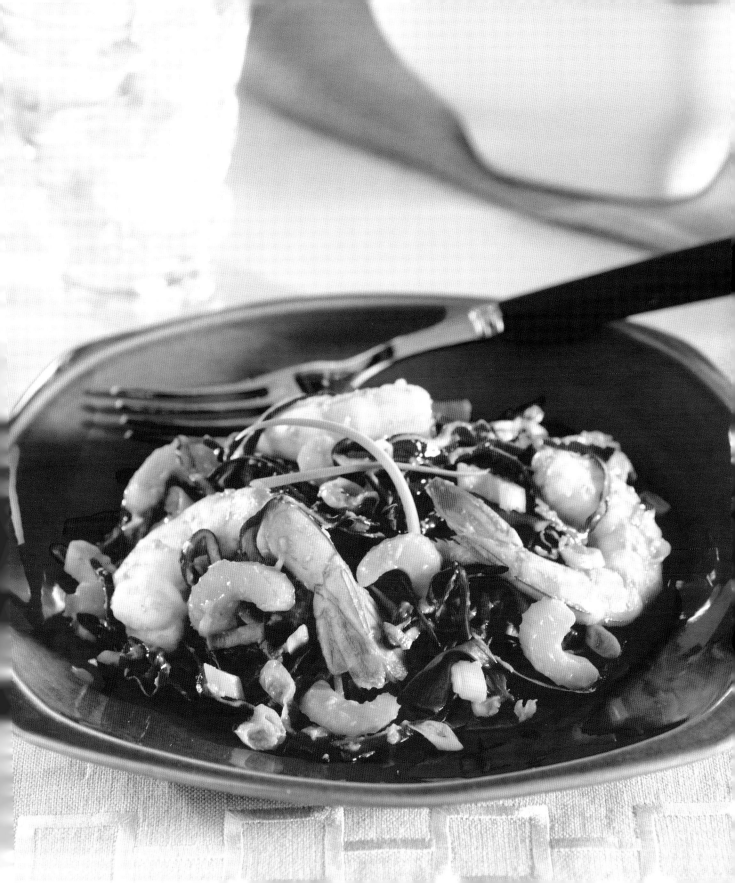

GRILLED TRI-COLORED PEPPER SALAD

makes 4 to 6 servings

1 *each* large red, yellow and green bell pepper, cut into halves or quarters

⅓ cup extra virgin olive oil

3 tablespoons balsamic vinegar

2 cloves garlic, minced

¼ teaspoon salt

¼ teaspoon black pepper

⅓ cup crumbled goat cheese (about 1½ ounces)

¼ cup thinly sliced fresh basil leaves

1 Prepare grill for direct cooking.

2 Place bell peppers, skin side down, on grid. Grill, covered, over high heat 10 to 12 minutes or until skin is charred. Transfer to paper bag. Close bag; let stand 10 to 15 minutes. Remove and discard skin. Place bell peppers in shallow serving dish.

3 Whisk oil, vinegar, garlic, salt and black pepper in small bowl until well blended. Pour over bell peppers; turn to coat. Let stand 30 minutes at room temperature. (Or cover and refrigerate up to 24 hours. Bring bell peppers to room temperature before serving.)

4 Sprinkle with cheese and basil just before serving.

PER SERVING:
calories 231, *total fat* 21g, *carbs* 9g, *net carbs* 7g, *dietary fiber* 2g, *protein* 3g

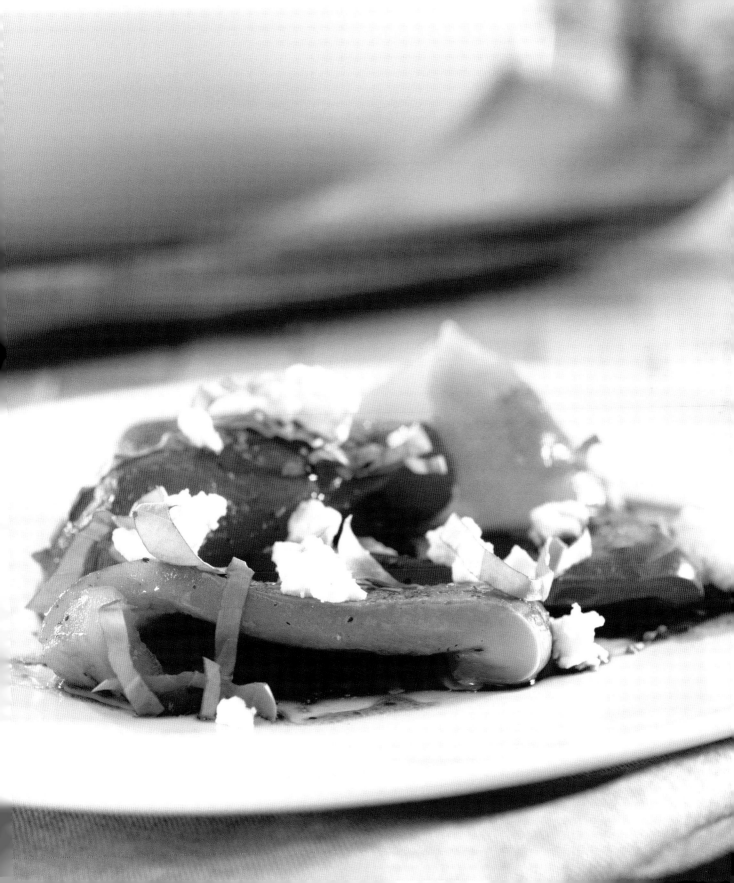

BLT CHICKEN SALAD FOR TWO

makes 2 servings

2 boneless skinless chicken breasts

¼ cup mayonnaise

½ teaspoon black pepper

4 large lettuce leaves

1 large tomato, seeded and diced

3 slices bacon, crisp-cooked and crumbled

1 hard-cooked egg, chopped

Additional mayonnaise (optional)

1 Prepare grill for direct cooking. Brush chicken with ¼ cup mayonnaise; sprinkle with pepper.

2 Grill chicken over medium heat 5 to 7 minutes per side or until no longer pink in center. Cool slightly; cut into thin strips.

3 Arrange lettuce on serving plates; top with chicken, tomato, bacon and egg. Serve with additional mayonnaise, if desired.

PER SERVING:

calories 426, *total fat* 30g, *carbs* 5g, *net carbs* 4g, *dietary fiber* 1g, *protein* 34g

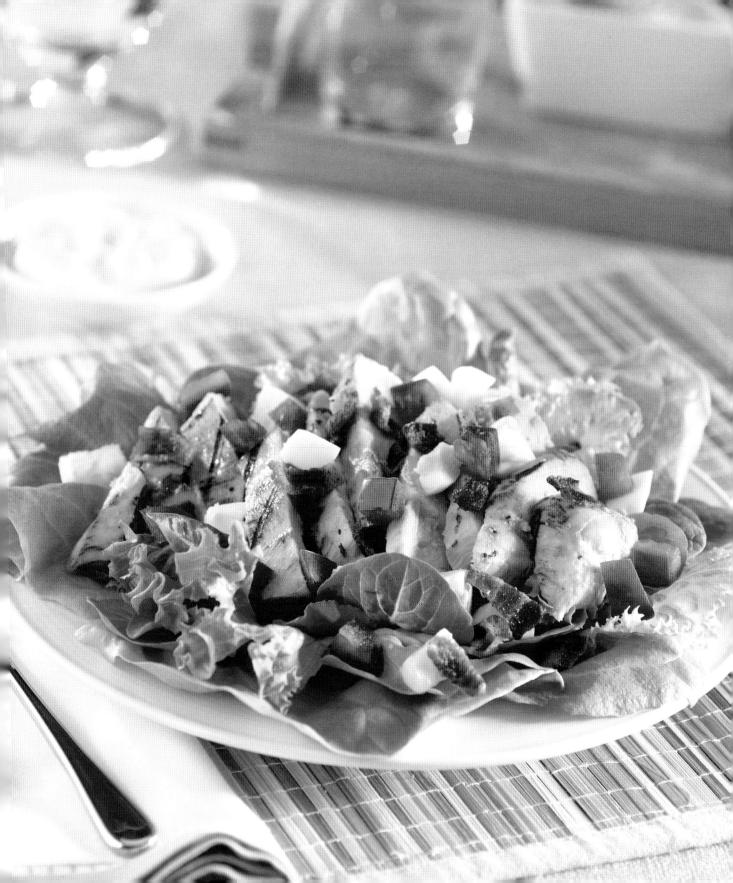

TOMATO, AVOCADO AND CUCUMBER SALAD

makes 4 servings

1½ tablespoons extra virgin olive oil

1 tablespoon balsamic vinegar

1 clove garlic, minced

¼ teaspoon salt

¼ teaspoon black pepper

2 cups diced seeded plum tomatoes

1 small ripe avocado, cut into ½-inch chunks

½ cup chopped cucumber

⅓ cup crumbled reduced-fat feta cheese

4 large red leaf lettuce leaves

Chopped fresh basil (optional)

1 Whisk oil, vinegar, garlic, salt and pepper in medium bowl until well blended. Add tomatoes and avocado; toss gently to coat. Stir in cucumber and cheese.

2 Arrange lettuce leaf on each serving plate. Spoon salad evenly onto lettuce leaves. Top with basil, if desired.

PER SERVING:

calories 180, *total fat* 10g, *carbs* 7g, *net carbs* 5g, *dietary fiber* 2g, *protein* 16g

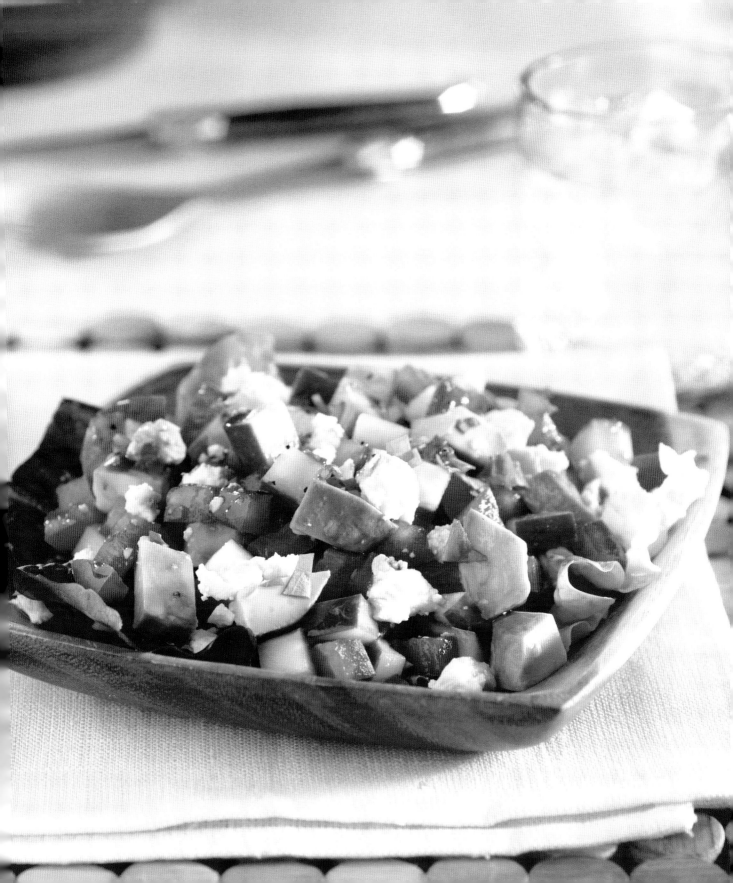

GREEN GODDESS COBB SALAD

makes 6 servings

Pickled Onions

- 1 cup thinly sliced red onion
- ½ cup white wine vinegar
- ¼ cup water
- 1 teaspoon salt

Dressing

- 1 cup mayonnaise
- 1 cup fresh Italian parsley leaves
- 1 cup baby arugula
- ¼ cup extra virgin olive oil
- 3 tablespoons lemon juice
- 3 tablespoons minced fresh chives
- 2 tablespoons fresh tarragon leaves

- 1 clove garlic, minced
- 1 teaspoon Dijon mustard
- ½ teaspoon salt
- ⅛ teaspoon black pepper

Salad

- 4 eggs
- 4 cups Italian salad blend (romaine and radicchio)
- 2 cups chopped stemmed kale
- 2 cups baby arugula
- 2 avocados, sliced and halved
- 2 tomatoes, cut into wedges
- 2 cups cooked chicken strips
- 1 cup chopped crisp-cooked bacon

1 For pickled onions, combine onion, vinegar, ¼ cup water and 1 teaspoon salt in large glass jar. Seal jar; shake well. Refrigerate at least 1 hour or up to 1 week.

2 For dressing, combine mayonnaise, parsley, 1 cup arugula, oil, lemon juice, chives, tarragon, garlic, mustard, ½ teaspoon salt and pepper in blender or food processor; blend until smooth, stopping to scrape down side once or twice. Transfer to jar; refrigerate until ready to use. Just before serving, thin dressing with 1 to 2 tablespoons water, if necessary, to reach desired consistency.

3 Fill medium saucepan with water; bring to a boil over high heat. Carefully lower eggs into water. Reduce heat to medium; boil gently 12 minutes. Drain eggs; add cold water and ice cubes to saucepan to cool eggs. When eggs are cool enough to handle, peel and cut into halves or quarters.

4 For salad, combine salad blend, kale, 2 cups arugula and pickled onions in large bowl; divide among six individual serving bowls. Top each salad with avocados, tomatoes, chicken, bacon and eggs. Top with dressing; toss to coat.

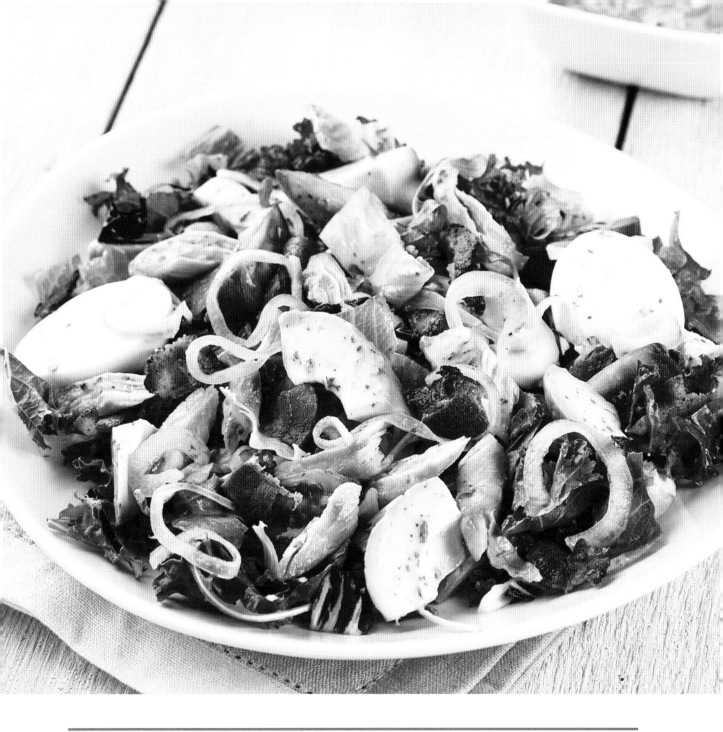

PER SERVING:
calories 1130, *total fat* 92g, *carbs* 21g, *net carbs* 11g, *dietary fiber* 10g, *protein* 60g

WEDGE SALAD

makes 4 servings

Dressing

- ¾ cup mayonnaise
- ½ cup buttermilk
- 1 cup crumbled blue cheese, divided
- 1 clove garlic, minced
- ⅛ teaspoon onion powder
- ⅛ teaspoon salt
- ⅛ teaspoon black pepper

Salad

- 1 head iceberg lettuce
- 1 large tomato, diced (about 1 cup)
- ½ small red onion, cut into thin rings
- ½ cup crumbled crisp-cooked bacon

1 For dressing, combine mayonnaise, buttermilk, ½ cup cheese, garlic, onion powder, salt and pepper in food processor or blender; process until smooth.

2 For salad, cut lettuce into quarters through stem end; remove stem from each wedge. Place wedges on individual serving plates; top with dressing. Sprinkle with tomato, onion, remaining ½ cup cheese and bacon.

PER SERVING:

calories 460, *total fat* 42g, *carbs* 9g, *net carbs* 7g, *dietary fiber* 2g, *protein* 13g

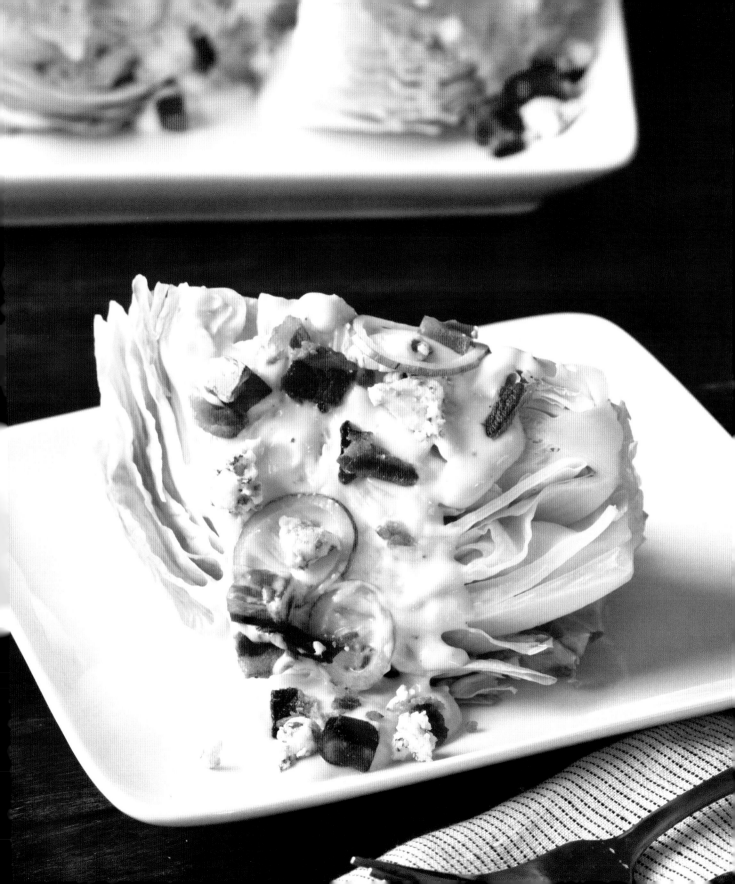

GRILLED CHICKEN CAPRESE SALAD

makes 2 servings

3 tablespoons extra virgin olive oil

2 tablespoons red wine vinegar

2 tablespoons chopped fresh basil

1 clove garlic, minced

1 teaspoon Dijon mustard

½ teaspoon salt

¼ teaspoon black pepper

⅔ cup cherry tomatoes, quartered

1 cup small fresh mozzarella cheese balls, quartered

2 boneless skinless chicken breasts (4 to 6 ounces each)

4 cups chopped romaine lettuce

2 avocados, halved

Additional fresh basil leaves for garnish

1 Prepare grill for direct cooking. Oil grid.

2 Whisk oil, vinegar, chopped basil, garlic, mustard, salt and pepper in medium bowl until well blended. Reserve 2 tablespoons mixture in small bowl.

3 Add tomatoes and cheese to medium bowl with oil mixture; toss gently to coat. Set aside while preparing chicken.

4 Brush half of reserved oil mixture over both sides of chicken. Grill chicken over medium-high heat about 5 minutes per side or until no longer pink in center.* Remove chicken to cutting board; let stand 5 minutes before slicing.

5 Slice chicken. Divide romaine among two serving bowls; top with chicken, tomato mixture and avocado halves. Brush remaining oil mixture over avocados. Garnish with basil leaves.

Or use stovetop grill pan sprayed with nonstick cooking spray.

PER SERVING:

calories 830, *total fat* 68g, *carbs* 24g, *net carbs* 8g, *dietary fiber* 16g, *protein* 42g

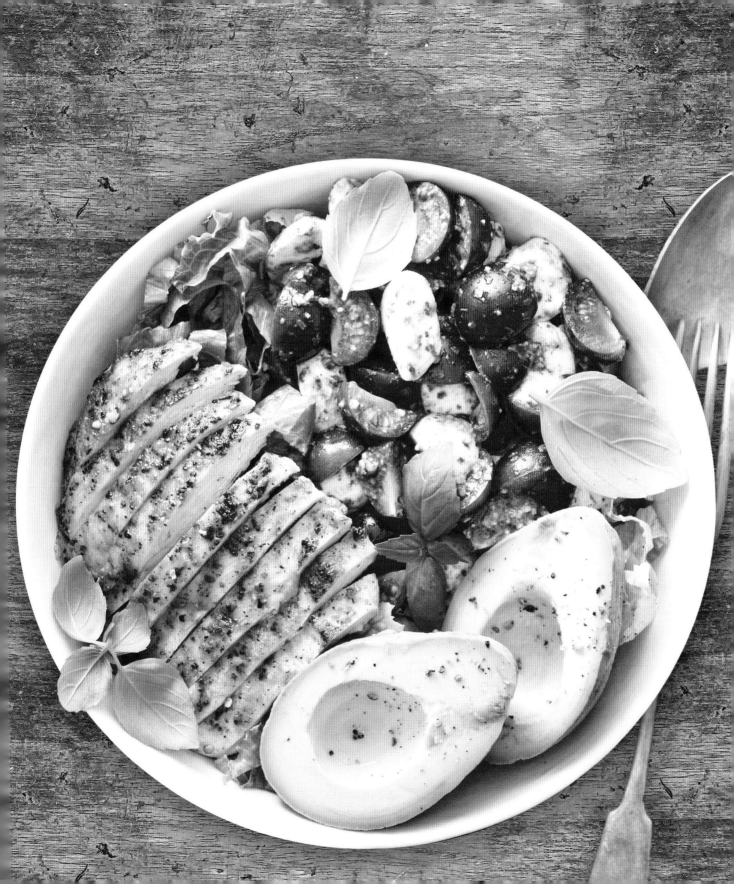

MARINATED TOMATO SALAD

makes 8 servings

1½ cups white wine or tarragon vinegar

½ teaspoon salt

¼ cup finely chopped shallots

2 tablespoons finely chopped fresh chives

2 tablespoons lemon juice

¼ teaspoon white pepper

2 tablespoons extra virgin olive oil

6 plum tomatoes, quartered

2 large yellow tomatoes,* sliced horizontally into ½-inch-thick slices

16 red cherry tomatoes, halved

16 small yellow pear tomatoes,* halved (optional)

Sunflower sprouts (optional)

Or substitute 10 plum tomatoes, quartered, for yellow tomatoes and yellow pear tomatoes.

1 Combine vinegar and salt in large bowl; stir until salt is completely dissolved. Add shallots, chives, lemon juice and pepper; mix well. Slowly whisk in oil until well blended.

2 Add tomatoes to marinade; toss gently to coat. Cover and let stand at room temperature 30 minutes or up to 2 hours before serving. Garnish with sunflower sprouts.

PER SERVING:

calories 60, *total fat* 4g, *carbs* 6g, *net carbs* 4g, *dietary fiber* 2g, *protein* 1g

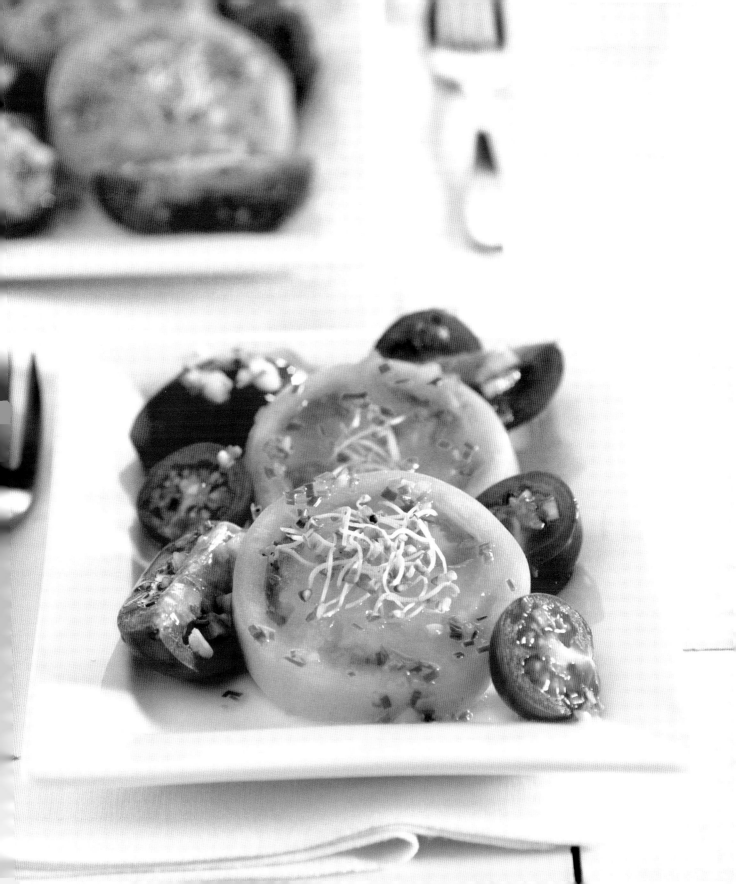

GAZPACHO SHRIMP SALAD

makes 4 servings

½ cup chunky salsa

1 tablespoon extra virgin olive oil

1 tablespoon balsamic vinegar

1 clove garlic, minced

8 cups torn mixed salad greens or romaine lettuce

1 large tomato, chopped

1 small ripe avocado, diced

½ cup thinly sliced unpeeled cucumber

8 ounces large cooked shrimp, peeled and deveined

½ cup chopped fresh cilantro

1 Combine salsa, oil, vinegar and garlic in small bowl; mix well.

2 Combine greens, tomato, avocado and cucumber in large bowl; toss gently. Divide salad among four serving plates; top with shrimp. Drizzle dressing over salads; sprinkle with cilantro.

PER SERVING:

calories 190, *total fat* 11g, *carbs* 10g, *net carbs* 5g, *dietary fiber* 5g, *protein* 14g

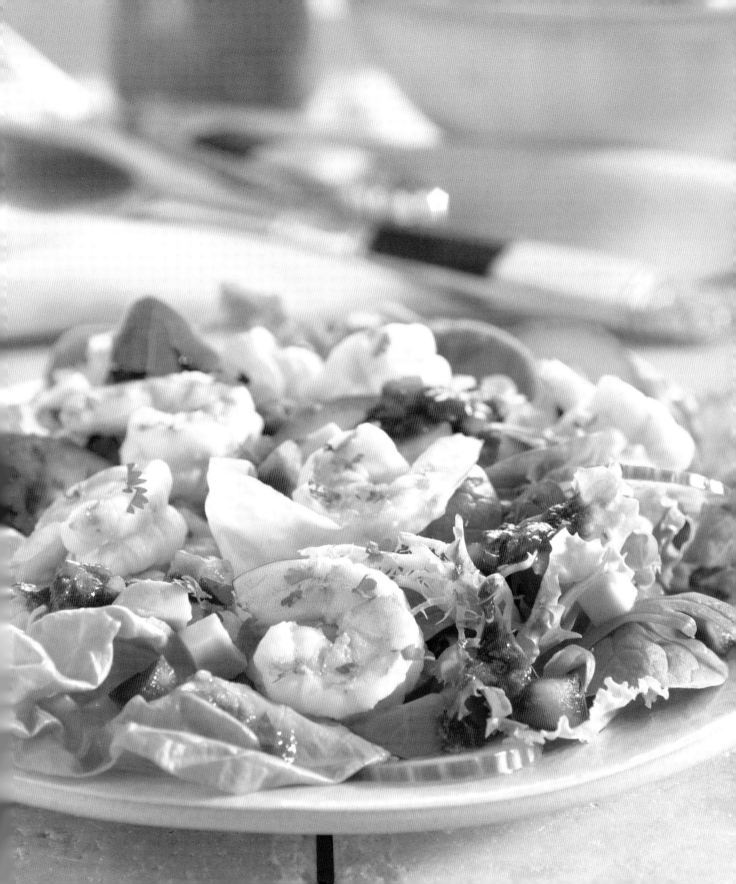

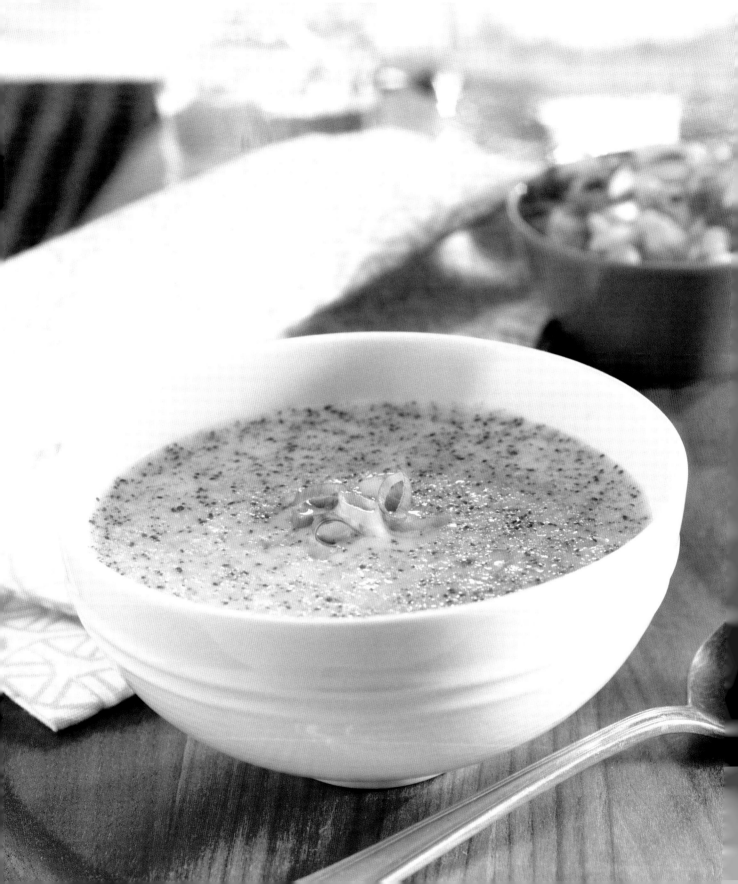

SOUPS

BROCCOLI CREAM SOUP

makes 5 servings

1 tablespoon olive oil

1½ cups chopped onions

1 pound fresh or frozen broccoli florets or spears

2 cups chicken or vegetable broth

6 tablespoons cream cheese

1 cup whole milk

¾ teaspoon salt

⅛ teaspoon ground red pepper

Thinly sliced green onions (optional)

1 Heat oil in large saucepan over medium-high heat. Add onions; cook and stir 4 minutes or until translucent. Add broccoli and broth; bring to a boil. Reduce heat to medium-low; cover and cook 10 minutes or until broccoli is tender.

2 Working in batches, process mixture in food processor or blender until smooth. (Or use hand-held immersion blender.) Return mixture to saucepan; heat over medium heat.

3 Whisk in cream cheese until melted. Stir in milk, salt and red pepper; cook 2 minutes or until heated through. Garnish with green onions.

PER SERVING:

calories 150, *total fat* 10g, *carbs* 13g, *net carbs* 10g, *dietary fiber* 3g, *protein* 6g

CHUNKY TOMATO-BASIL SOUP

makes 6 servings

2 tablespoons olive oil

1 cup chopped onion

2 cloves garlic, minced

5 cups fresh tomatoes, peeled, seeded and chopped, divided

1 can (6 ounces) tomato paste

1½ teaspoons dried basil

¼ teaspoon salt

½ teaspoon dried oregano

¼ teaspoon black pepper

4 cups reduced-sodium chicken broth

1 Heat oil in large saucepan over medium heat. Add onion and garlic; cover and cook 7 minutes or until onion is tender, stirring occasionally.

2 Reserve 1 cup fresh tomatoes; add remaining tomatoes to saucepan. Add tomato paste, basil, salt, oregano and pepper; cook and stir 1 minute. Stir in broth; bring to a boil. Reduce heat to low; cover and cook 30 minutes.

3 Pour about one third of hot soup into blender; blend until smooth. (Or use hand-held immersion blender.) Repeat with remaining soup, one third at a time. Return puréed soup to saucepan; stir in reserved tomatoes. Cook until heated through.

PER SERVING:

calories 110, *total fat* 5g, *carbs* 13g, *net carbs* 10g, *dietary fiber* 3g, *protein* 4g

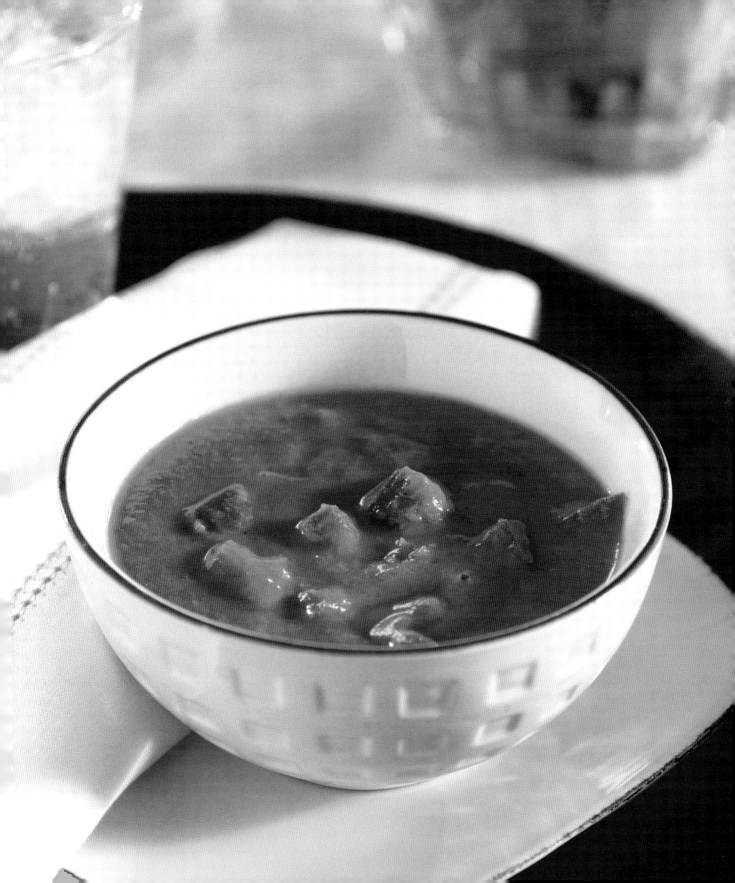

CREAM OF AVOCADO SOUP

makes 12 servings

6 medium avocados, cut into halves and pitted

Lemon juice

2 cups vegetable broth, divided

4 eggs*

4 cups whole milk, divided

½ teaspoon salt

¼ teaspoon white pepper

3 cups sour cream, divided

Black caviar and ground red pepper (optional)

Use clean, uncracked eggs.

1 Scoop out flesh of avocados leaving ¼-inch shell; set aside avocado flesh. Lightly sprinkle shells with lemon juice to prevent browning. Cover and refrigerate shells until ready to serve.

2 Combine avocado flesh and 1 cup broth in small batches in food processor or blender; process until smooth. Transfer to large bowl; set aside.

3 Beat eggs and 2 cups milk in top of double boiler. Heat slowly over hot, not boiling, water; stir until mixture is thick enough to coat back of spoon. Remove from heat; stir in remaining 1 cup broth. Let stand at room temperature until cool.

4 Stir cooled egg mixture, salt and white pepper into avocado mixture. Stir in 2 cups sour cream until smooth. Stir in remaining 2 cups milk. Process soup in small batches in food processor or blender until smooth. Add additional salt and white pepper if necessary. Cover and refrigerate until very cold.

5 To serve, pour cold soup into avocado shells. Top each portion with dollop of sour cream. Garnish, if desired.

PER SERVING:

calories 360, *total fat* 31g, *carbs* 15g, *net carbs* 8g, *dietary fiber* 7g, *protein* 9g

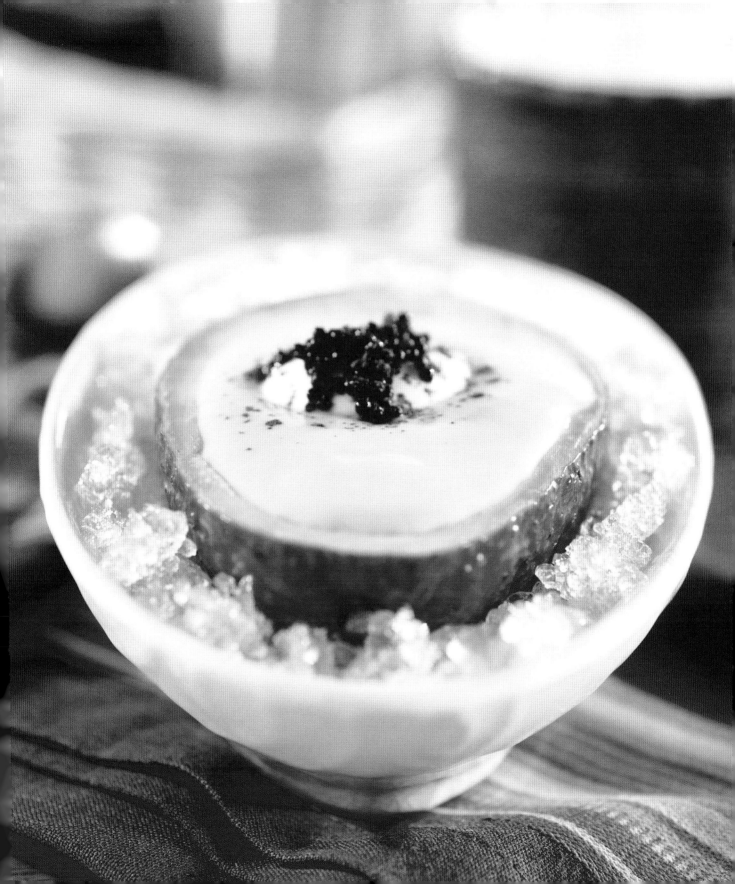

SPICY THAI SHRIMP SOUP

makes 4 servings

1 tablespoon vegetable oil

1 pound medium raw shrimp, peeled and deveined, shells reserved

1 jalapeño pepper,* cut into slivers

1 tablespoon paprika

¼ teaspoon ground red pepper

4 cans (about 14 ounces each) chicken broth

1 (½-inch) strip *each* lemon and lime peel

1 can (15 ounces) straw mushrooms, drained

Juice of 1 lemon

Juice of 1 lime

2 tablespoons soy sauce

1 red Thai pepper* or red jalapeño pepper* *or* ¼ small red bell pepper, cut into strips

¼ cup fresh cilantro leaves

*Chile peppers can sting and irritate the skin, so wear rubber gloves when handling peppers and do not touch your eyes.

1 Heat large skillet over medium-high heat 1 minute. Add oil; heat 30 seconds. Add shrimp and jalapeño; cook and stir 1 minute. Add paprika and ground red pepper; cook and stir 1 minute or until shrimp are pink and opaque. Transfer shrimp mixture to medium bowl.

2 Add shrimp shells to skillet; cook and stir 30 seconds. Add broth and lemon and lime peels; bring to a boil. Reduce heat to low; cover and cook 15 minutes.

3 Remove shells and peels with slotted spoon; discard. Add mushrooms and shrimp mixture to broth; bring to a boil over medium heat. Stir in lemon and lime juices, soy sauce and Thai pepper; cook until heated through. Sprinkle with cilantro. Serve immediately.

PER SERVING:

calories 200, *total fat* 7g, *carbs* 6g, *net carbs* 4g, *dietary fiber* 2g, *protein* 14g

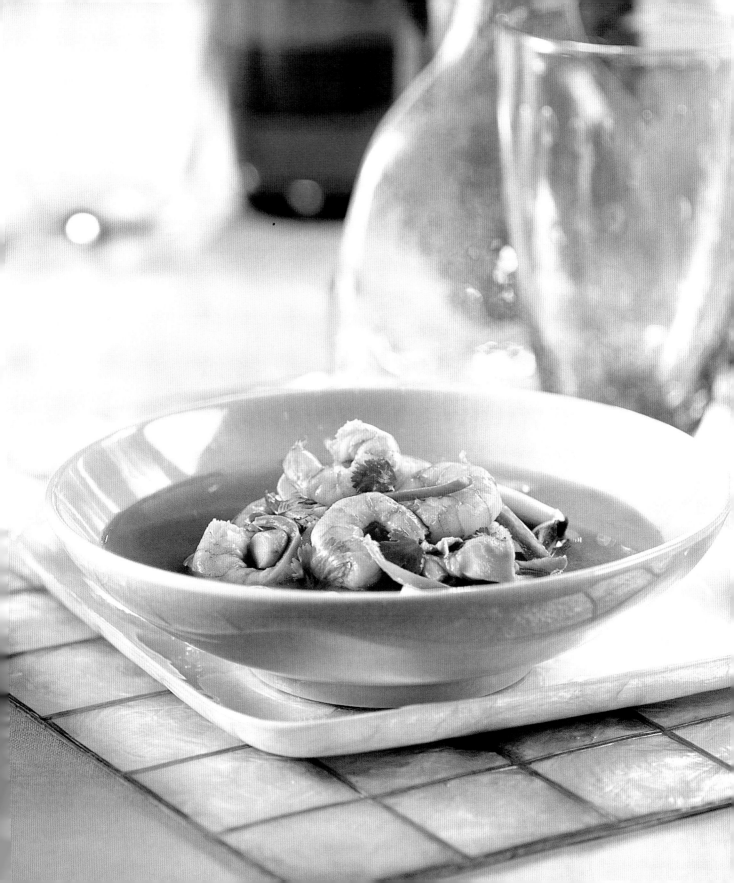

COLD YOGURT SOUP

makes 4 servings

1 cup finely chopped cooked chicken

1 teaspoon lemon juice

¾ teaspoon minced fresh dill *or* ¼ teaspoon dried dill weed

½ teaspoon salt

⅛ teaspoon garlic powder

Pinch white pepper

2 cups plain whole milk yogurt

1 small cucumber, seeded and diced

⅓ cup chopped celery

3 tablespoons thinly sliced green onions

1 Combine chicken, lemon juice, dill, salt, garlic powder and pepper in small bowl; mix well. Cover and refrigerate 30 minutes.

2 Place yogurt in medium bowl; stir with fork or whisk until smooth and creamy. Add chicken mixture, cucumber, celery and green onions to yogurt; stir gently to coat.

PER SERVING:

calories 150, *total fat* 6g, *carbs* 10g, *net carbs* 9g, *dietary fiber* 1g, *protein* 13g

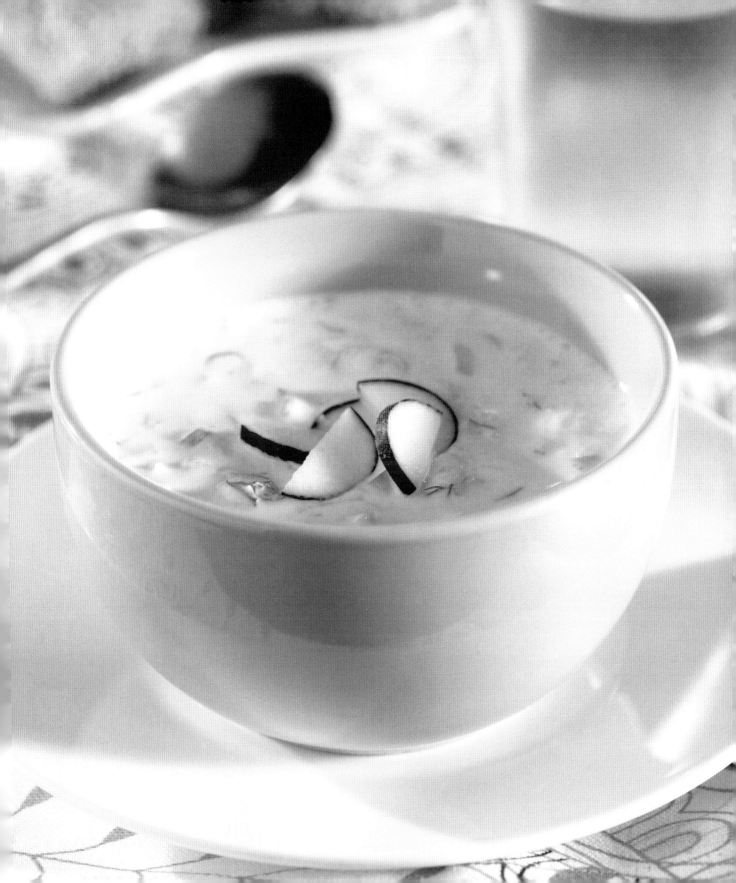

ROMAN SPINACH SOUP

makes 8 servings

6 cups reduced-sodium chicken broth

1 cup liquid egg substitute *or 4 eggs*, beaten

¼ cup minced fresh basil

3 tablespoons grated Parmesan cheese

2 tablespoons lemon juice

1 tablespoon minced fresh parsley

¼ teaspoon white pepper

⅛ teaspoon ground nutmeg

8 cups packed fresh spinach, chopped

Fresh lemon slices (optional)

1 Bring broth to a boil in large saucepan over medium heat.

2 Beat egg substitute, basil, cheese, lemon juice, parsley, white pepper and nutmeg in medium bowl until well blended.

3 Stir spinach into broth; cook 1 minute. Slowly pour egg mixture into broth mixture, whisking constantly so egg threads form. Cook 2 to 3 minutes or until egg is cooked. (Soup may look curdled.) Garnish with lemon slices. Serve immediately.

PER SERVING:

calories 46, *total fat* 1g, *carbs* 4g, *net carbs* 3g, *dietary fiber* 1g, *protein* 6g

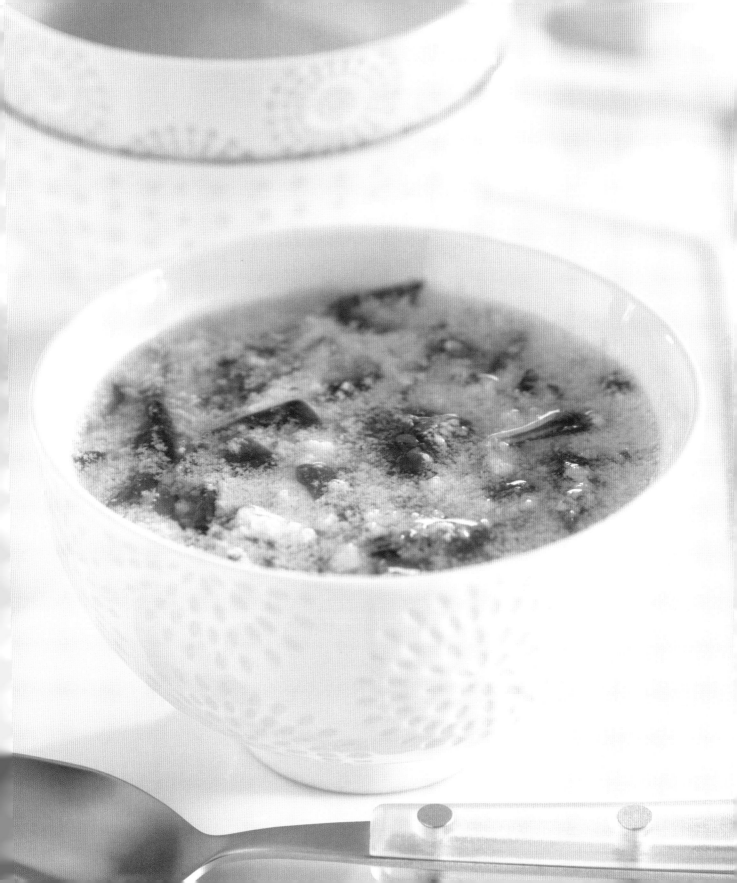

BEEFY BROCCOLI
AND CHEESE SOUP

makes 4 servings

¼ pound ground beef

2 cups beef broth

1 bag (10 ounces) frozen chopped broccoli, thawed

¼ cup chopped onion

1 cup whole milk

1 cup (4 ounces) shredded sharp Cheddar cheese

1½ teaspoons chopped fresh oregano *or* ½ teaspoon dried oregano

Salt and black pepper

Hot pepper sauce

1 Brown beef in large skillet over medium-high heat 6 to 8 minutes, stirring to break up meat. Drain fat.

2 Pour broth into medium saucepan; bring to a boil over medium-high heat. Add broccoli and onion; cook 5 minutes or until broccoli is tender. Stir in milk and beef; cook until thickened and heated through, stirring frequently.

3 Add cheese and oregano; stir until cheese is melted. Season with salt, black pepper and hot pepper sauce.

PER SERVING:

calories 260, *total fat* 16g, *carbs* 8g, *net carbs* 6g, *dietary fiber* 2g, *protein* 19g

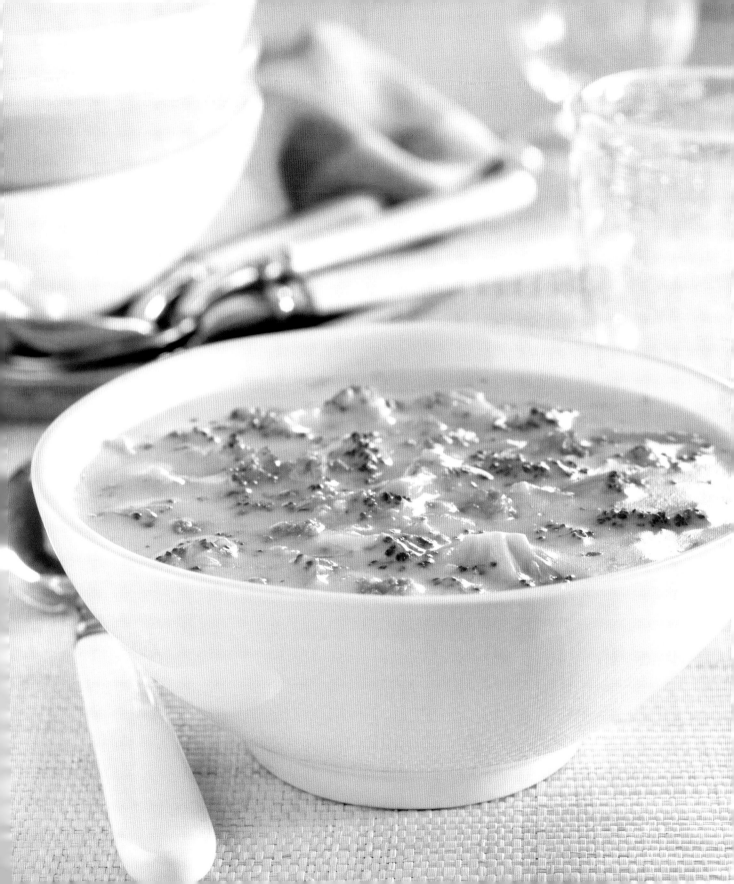

CIOPPINO

makes 4 servings

1 teaspoon olive oil

1 large onion, chopped

1 cup sliced celery (with celery tops)

1 clove garlic, minced

4 cups water

1 tablespoon Italian seasoning

1 fish-flavored bouillon cube

¼ pound cod or other boneless mild-flavored fish fillets, cut into ½-inch pieces

1 large tomato, chopped

1 can (10 ounces) baby clams, rinsed and drained (optional)

¼ pound small raw shrimp, peeled and deveined

¼ pound raw bay scallops

¼ cup flaked crabmeat or crabmeat blend

2 tablespoons lemon juice

1 Heat oil in large saucepan over medium heat. Add onion, celery and garlic; cook and stir 5 minutes or until onion is soft.

2 Add water, Italian seasoning and bouillon; bring to a boil over high heat. Stir in fish and tomato. Reduce heat to medium-low; cook about 5 minutes or until fish is opaque.

3 Add clams, if desired, shrimp, scallops, crabmeat and lemon juice; cook about 5 minutes or until shrimp and scallops are opaque.

PER SERVING:

calories 122, *total fat* 2g, *carbs* 8g, *net carbs* 6g, *dietary fiber* 2g, *protein* 18g

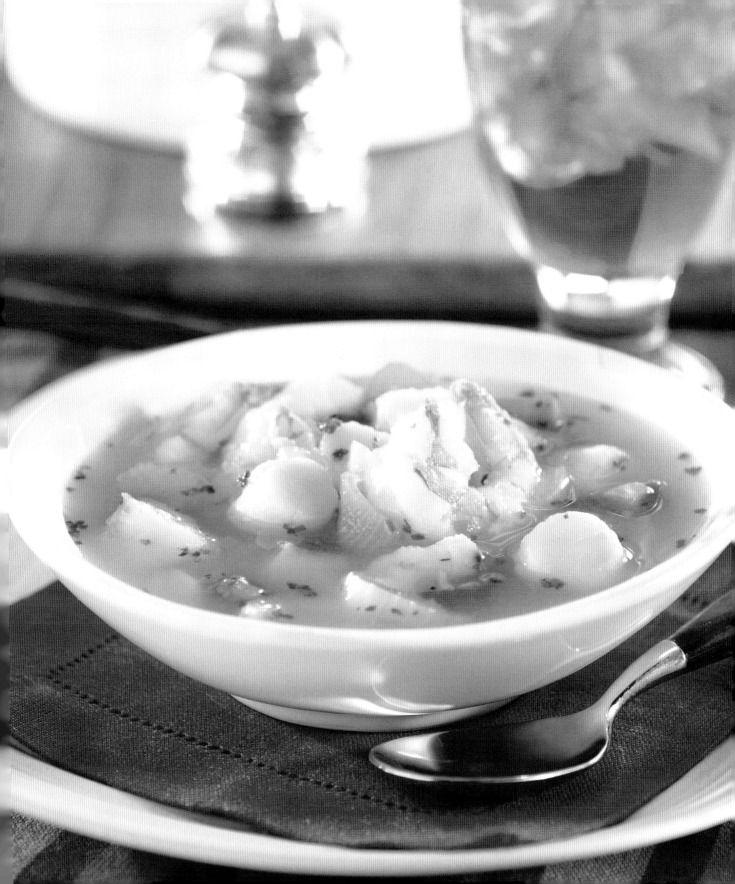

CHILLED CUCUMBER SOUP

makes 4 servings

1 large cucumber, peeled and coarsely chopped

¾ cup reduced-fat sour cream

¼ cup packed fresh dill

½ teaspoon salt (optional)

⅛ teaspoon white pepper (optional)

1½ cups reduced-sodium chicken or vegetable broth

Fresh dill sprigs (optional)

1 Place cucumber in food processor; process until finely chopped. Add sour cream, ¼ cup dill, salt and white pepper, if desired; process until almost smooth.

2 Transfer mixture to large bowl; stir in broth. Cover and refrigerate at least 2 hours or up to 24 hours. Garnish with dill sprigs.

PER SERVING:

calories 67, *total fat* 4g, *carbs* 6g, *net carbs* 5g, *dietary fiber* 1g, *protein* 3g

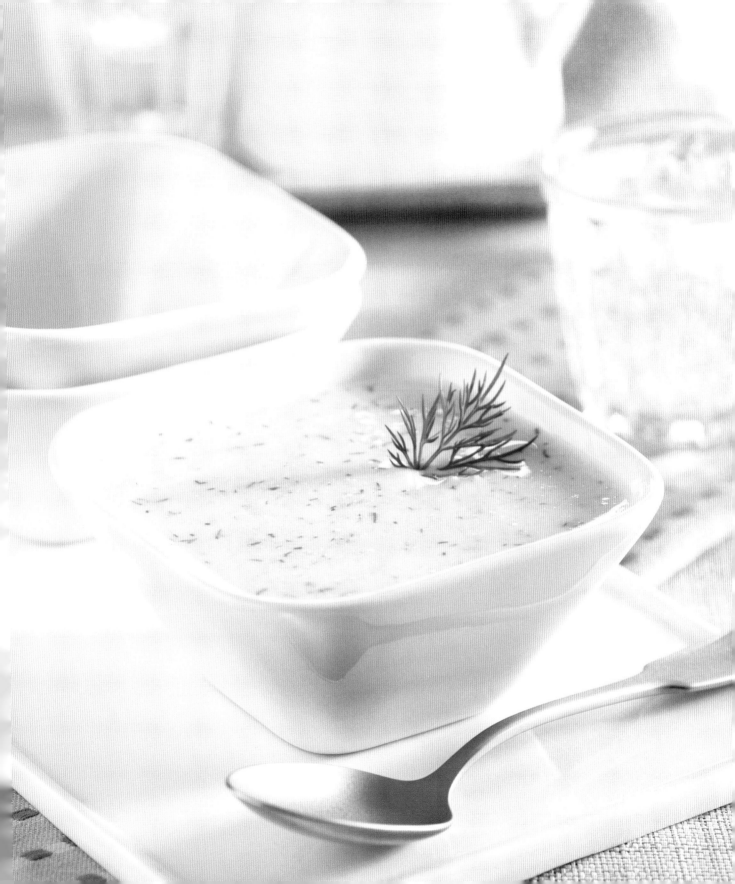

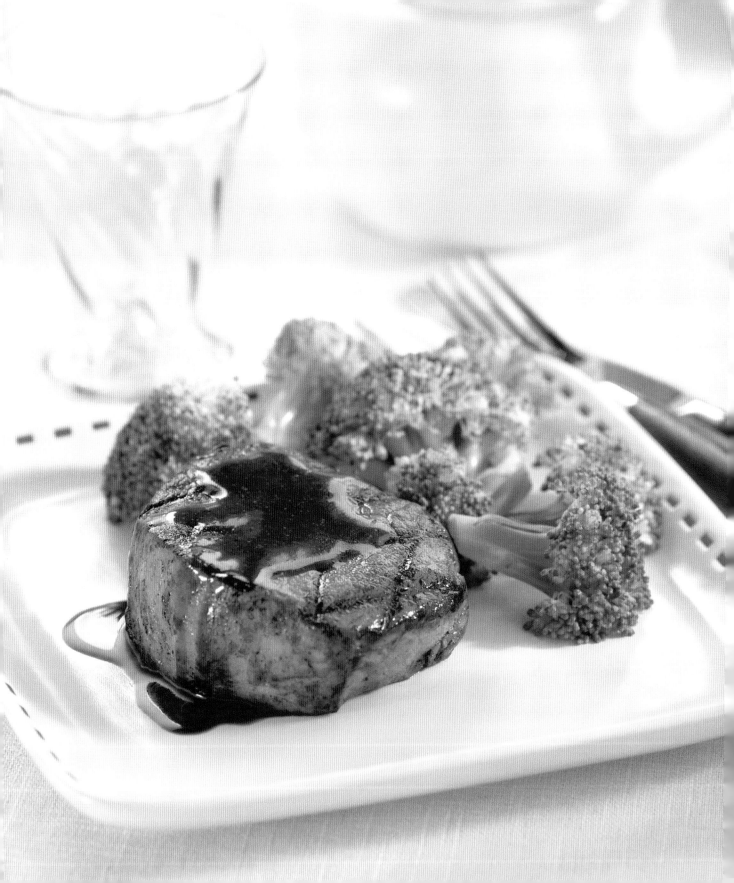

MEAT

BALSAMIC GRILLED PORK CHOPS

makes 2 servings

2 tablespoons balsamic vinegar

2 tablespoons soy sauce

1 teaspoon Dijon mustard

⅛ teaspoon red pepper flakes

2 boneless pork chops (4 ounces each)

1 Whisk vinegar, soy sauce, mustard and red pepper flakes in small bowl until well blended. Reserve 1 tablespoon marinade; refrigerate until ready to serve.

2 Place pork in large resealable food storage bag; pour remaining marinade over pork. Seal bag; turn to coat. Marinate in refrigerator 2 hours or up to 24 hours.

3 Spray grill pan with nonstick cooking spray; heat over medium-high heat. Remove pork from marinade; discard marinade. Cook pork 4 minutes per side or until barely pink in center. Drizzle with reserved 1 tablespoon marinade.

PER SERVING:

calories 180, *total fat* 5g, *carbs* 4g, *net carbs* 3g, *dietary fiber* 1g, *protein* 26g

FLANK STEAK WITH ITALIAN SALSA

makes 6 servings

2 tablespoons olive oil

2 teaspoons balsamic vinegar

1 flank steak (1½ pounds)

1 tablespoon minced garlic

¾ teaspoon salt, divided

¾ teaspoon black pepper, divided

1 cup diced plum tomatoes

⅓ cup chopped pitted kalamata olives

2 tablespoons chopped fresh basil

1 Whisk oil and vinegar in medium bowl until well blended. Place steak in shallow dish. Spread garlic over steak; sprinkle with ½ teaspoon salt and ½ teaspoon pepper. Spoon 2 tablespoons oil mixture over steak. Marinate in refrigerator at least 20 minutes or up to 2 hours.

2 Add tomatoes, olives, basil, remaining ¼ teaspoon salt and ¼ teaspoon pepper to remaining oil mixture in bowl; mix well.

3 Prepare grill for direct cooking or preheat broiler. Remove steak from marinade; discard marinade. (Leave garlic on steak.)

4 Grill steak over medium-high heat 5 to 6 minutes per side for medium rare. Remove to cutting board; tent with foil. Let stand 5 minutes before slicing. Cut steak diagonally into thin slices across the grain. Serve with tomato mixture.

PER SERVING:

calories 191, *total fat* 11g, *carbs* 4g, *net carbs* 3g, *dietary fiber* 1g, *protein* 18g

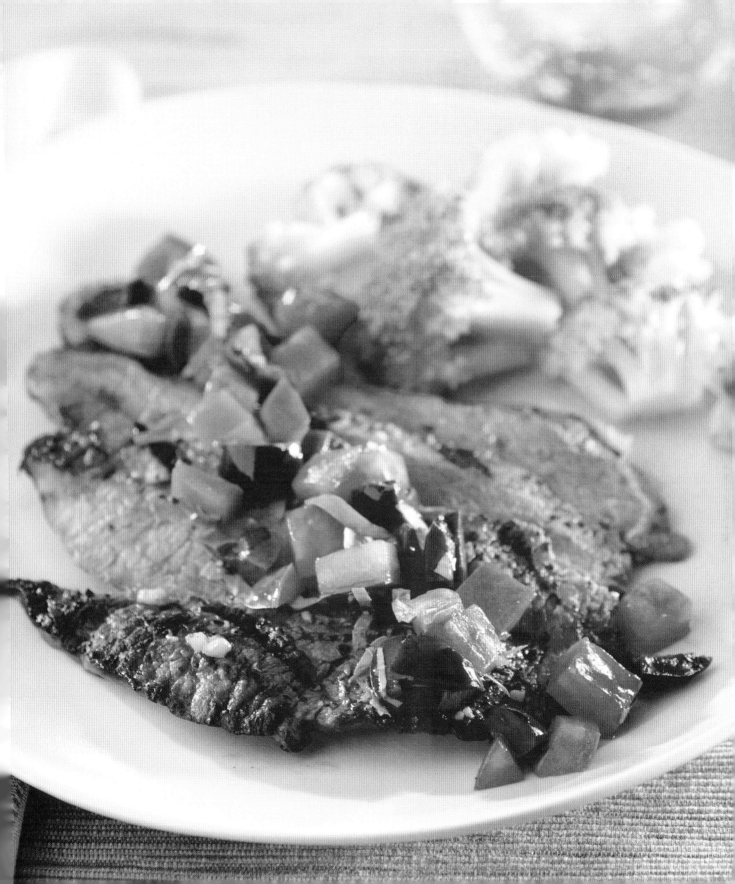

BEEF PATTIES WITH BLUE CHEESE AND SQUASH

makes 4 servings

1 pound lean ground beef

2 tablespoons steak sauce

½ teaspoon salt, divided

¼ cup crumbled blue cheese

1 teaspoon olive oil

8 ounces (about 1½ cups) yellow squash, cut in half lengthwise, then cut crosswise into ½-inch slices

1 medium onion, cut into 8 wedges

¼ cup finely chopped fresh parsley

1 Combine beef, steak sauce and ¼ teaspoon salt in small bowl; mix well. Shape into four patties.

2 Spray large nonstick skillet with nonstick cooking spray; heat over medium-high heat. Add patties; cook 4 minutes. Turn patties; cook over medium heat 3 to 4 minutes or until cooked through (160°F). Remove to plate. Sprinkle each patty with 1 tablespoon cheese; tent with foil.

3 Add oil to same skillet. Add squash and onion; cook 5 to 6 minutes over medium-high heat or until edges of vegetables begin to brown, stirring occasionally. Sprinkle with remaining ¼ teaspoon salt. Spoon vegetables over beef; sprinkle with parsley.

PER SERVING:

calories 219, *total fat* 9g, *carbs* 6g, *net carbs* 5g, *dietary fiber* 1g, *protein* 27g

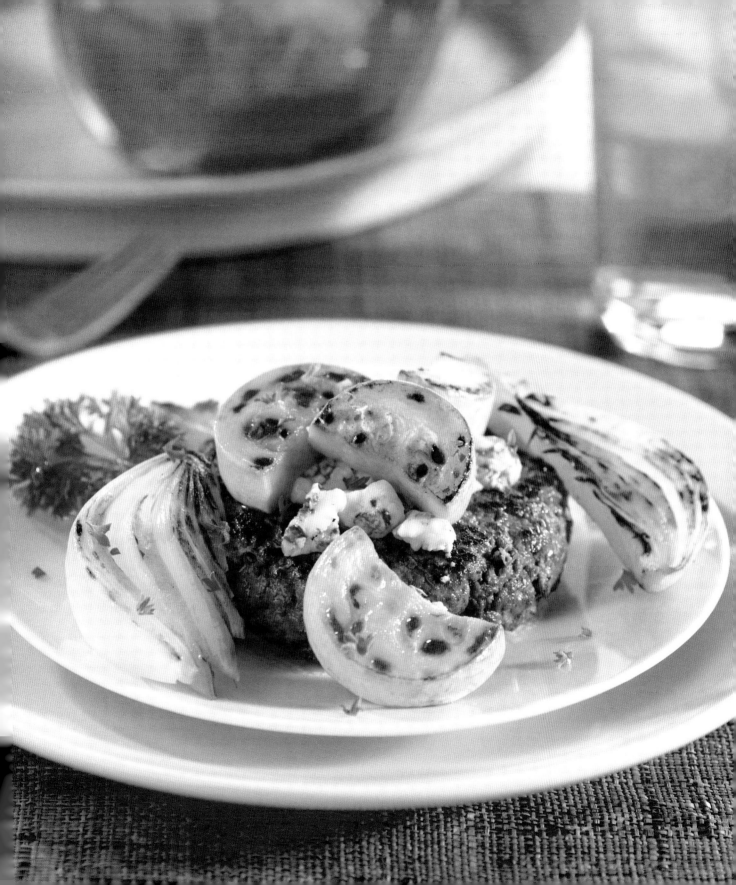

PORK CURRY OVER CAULIFLOWER COUSCOUS

makes 6 servings

3 tablespoons olive oil, divided

2 tablespoons mild curry powder

2 teaspoons minced garlic

1½ pounds boneless pork (shoulder, loin or chops), cubed

1 red or green bell pepper, diced

1 tablespoon cider vinegar

½ teaspoon salt

2 cups water

1 large head cauliflower

1 Heat 2 tablespoons oil in large saucepan over medium heat. Add curry powder and garlic; cook and stir 1 to 2 minutes or until garlic is golden.

2 Add pork; cook and stir 5 to 7 minutes or until barely pink in center. Add bell pepper and vinegar; cook and stir 3 minutes or until bell pepper is soft. Sprinkle with salt.

3 Stir in water; bring to a boil. Reduce heat to low; cook 30 to 45 minutes or until liquid is reduced and pork is tender, stirring occasionally. (Add additional water as needed.)

4 Meanwhile, trim and core cauliflower; cut into equal pieces. Place in food processor; pulse until cauliflower is in small uniform pieces about the size of cooked couscous. *Do not purée.*

5 Heat remaining 1 tablespoon oil in large nonstick skillet over medium heat. Add cauliflower; cook and stir 5 minutes or until crisp-tender. *Do not overcook.* Serve pork over cauliflower.

PER SERVING:

calories 267, *total fat* 15g, *carbs* 7g, *net carbs* 2g, *dietary fiber* 5g, *protein* 28g

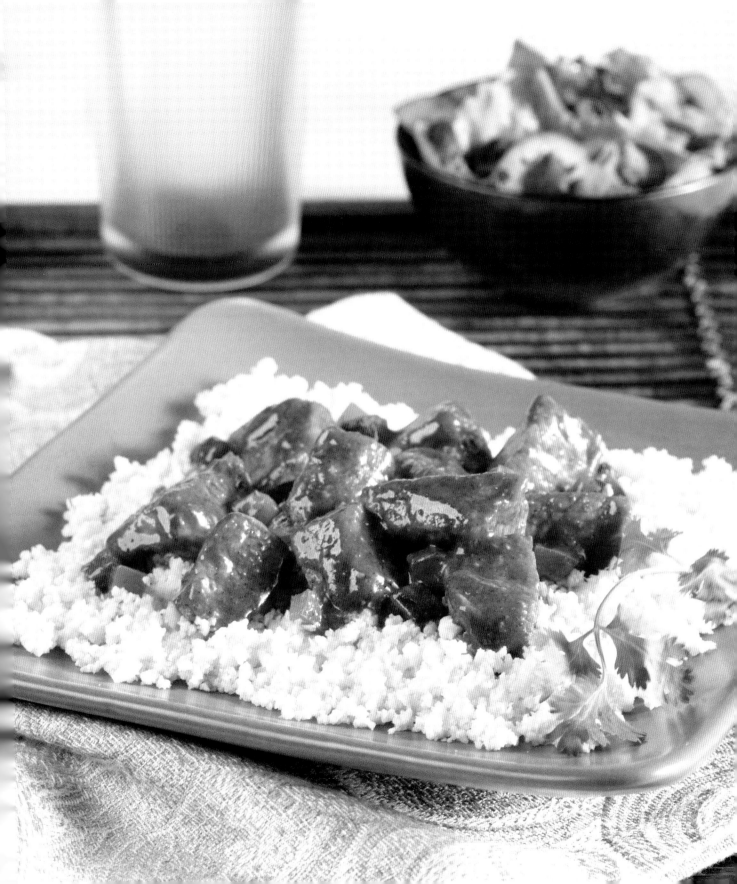

KOREAN BEEF SHORT RIBS

makes 6 servings

2½ pounds beef chuck flanken-style
    short ribs, cut ⅜ to ½ inch thick*

¼ cup chopped green onions

¼ cup water

¼ cup soy sauce

2 teaspoons grated fresh ginger

2 teaspoons dark sesame oil

2 cloves garlic, minced

½ teaspoon black pepper

1 tablespoon sesame seeds, toasted

**Flanken-style ribs can be ordered
from your butcher. They are cross-cut
short ribs sawed through the bones.*

1 Place ribs in large resealable food storage bag. Combine green onions, water, soy sauce, ginger, oil, garlic and pepper in small bowl; mix well. Pour mixture over ribs. Seal bag; turn to coat. Marinate in refrigerator at least 4 hours or up to 8 hours, turning occasionally.

2 Prepare grill for direct cooking. Remove ribs from marinade; reserve marinade.

3 Grill ribs, covered, over medium-high heat 5 minutes. Brush lightly with reserved marinade; turn and brush again. Discard remaining marinade. Grill, covered, 5 to 6 minutes for medium (165°F) or to desired doneness. Sprinkle with sesame seeds.

PER SERVING:

calories 417, *total fat* 24g, *carbs* 6g, *net carbs* 5g, *dietary fiber* 1g, *protein* 42g

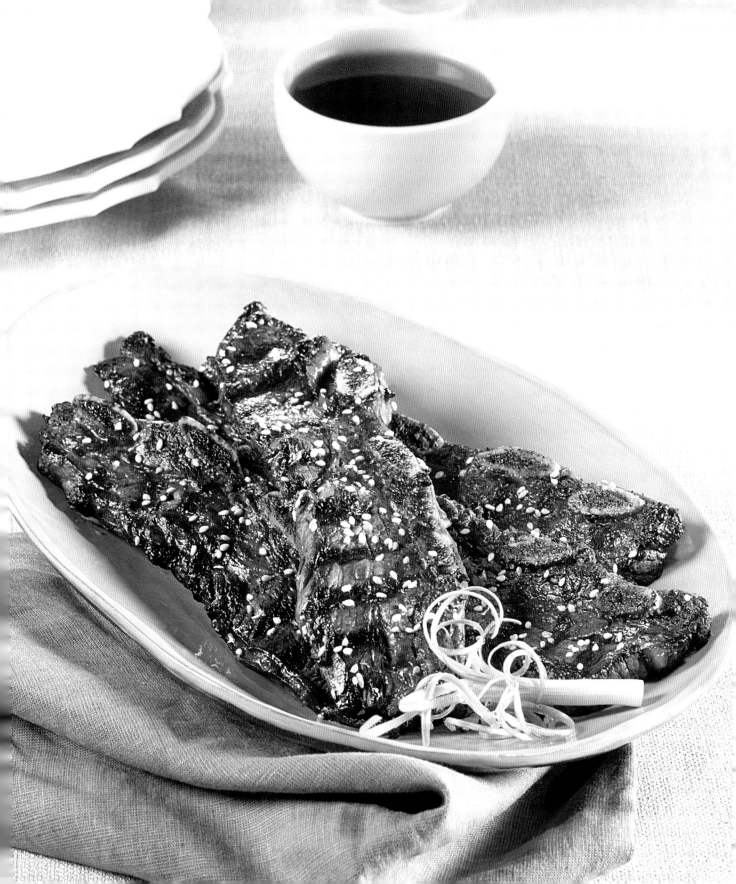

STUFFED EGGPLANT

makes 4 servings

2 eggplants (about 8 to 12 ounces each), halved lengthwise

1 teaspoon salt

1½ teaspoons chopped garlic

1 teaspoon black pepper

1 pound boneless beef sirloin steak, trimmed and cut into ¼-inch strips

2 cups sliced red and green bell peppers

2 cups sliced mushrooms

¼ cup water

Paprika (optional)

1 Preheat oven to 450°F. Spray baking dish with nonstick cooking spray.

2 Place eggplant halves cut sides up in large baking dish; pierce flesh with fork in about 8 places. Sprinkle each eggplant half with ¼ teaspoon salt. Cover with foil; bake 45 minutes.

3 Meanwhile, spray large nonstick skillet with cooking spray. Add garlic and black pepper; cook and stir over medium heat 2 minutes. Add beef; cook and stir 5 minutes. Add bell peppers; cook 5 minutes, stirring occasionally. Add mushrooms; cook 5 minutes, stirring occasionally. Stir in water; cover and remove from heat.

4 Remove eggplant from oven, let cool 5 minutes. Mash cooked eggplant centers with fork without breaking shells. Top each eggplant half with one fourth of beef mixture; stir into mashed eggplant.

5 Cover with foil; bake 15 minutes. Sprinkle with paprika, if desired.

PER SERVING:

calories 195, *total fat* 5g, *carbs* 12g, *net carbs* 8g, *dietary fiber* 4g, *protein* 25g

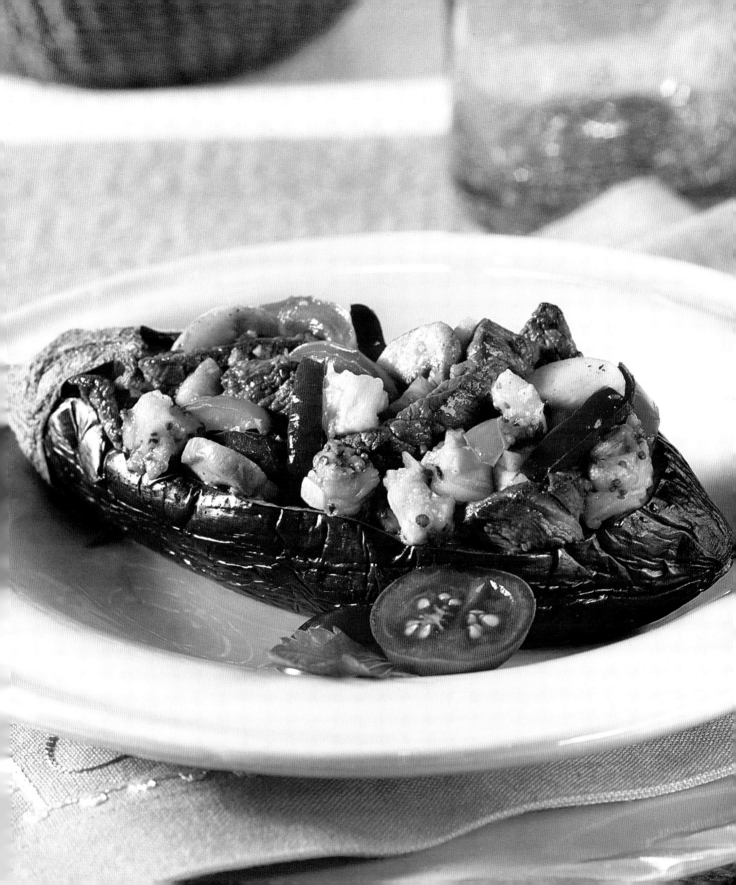

PORK TENDERLOIN WITH AVOCADO-TOMATILLO SALSA

makes 4 servings

1½ teaspoons chili powder

½ teaspoon ground cumin

1 pound pork tenderloin

1 teaspoon extra virgin olive oil

Salsa

2 medium tomatillos, husked and diced

½ ripe medium avocado, diced

1 jalapeño pepper,* seeded and finely chopped

1 clove garlic, minced

2 tablespoons finely chopped red onion

1 tablespoon lime juice

1 to 2 tablespoons chopped fresh cilantro

⅛ teaspoon salt

4 lime wedges (optional)

*Jalapeño peppers can sting and irritate the skin, so wear rubber gloves when handling and do not touch your eyes.

1 Preheat oven to 425°F. Line baking sheet with foil. Combine chili powder and cumin in small bowl; mix well. Sprinkle on all sides of pork, pressing to adhere.

2 Heat oil in large nonstick skillet over medium-high heat. Add pork; cook 3 minutes or until browned. Turn and cook 2 to 3 minutes or until well browned. Place on prepared baking sheet.

3 Bake 20 to 25 minutes or until pork is barely pink in center. Remove to cutting board; tent with foil. Let stand 5 minutes before slicing.

4 Combine salsa ingredients in small bowl; toss gently to blend. Slice pork; serve with salsa and lime wedges, if desired.

PER SERVING:

calories 174, *total fat* 6g, *carbs* 4g, *net carbs* 2g, *dietary fiber* 2g, *protein* 25g

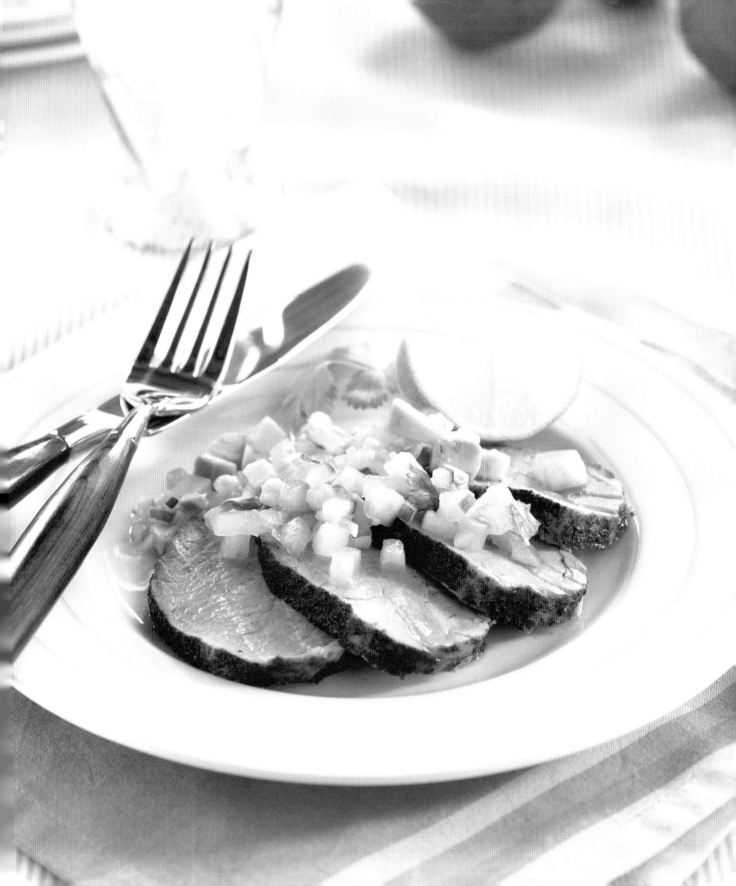

CHILI Á LA MEXICO

makes 6 servings

2 pounds ground beef

2 cups finely chopped onions

2 cloves garlic, minced

1 can (28 ounces) whole tomatoes, undrained and coarsely chopped

1 can (6 ounces) tomato paste

1½ to 2 tablespoons chili powder

1 teaspoon ground cumin

¼ teaspoon salt

¼ teaspoon ground red pepper

¼ teaspoon ground cloves (optional)

Lime wedges and fresh cilantro sprigs (optional)

1 Brown beef in deep skillet over medium-high heat 6 to 8 minutes, stirring to break up meat. Drain fat.

2 Add onions and garlic to skillet; cook and stir over medium heat 5 minutes or until onions are softened.

3 Stir in tomatoes with juice, tomato paste, chili powder, cumin, salt, ground red pepper and cloves, if desired; bring to a boil over high heat. Reduce heat to low; cover and cook 30 minutes, stirring occasionally. Garnish with lime wedges and cilantro.

PER SERVING:

calories 350, *total fat* 18g, *carbs* 16g, *net carbs* 11g, *dietary fiber* 5g, *protein* 30g

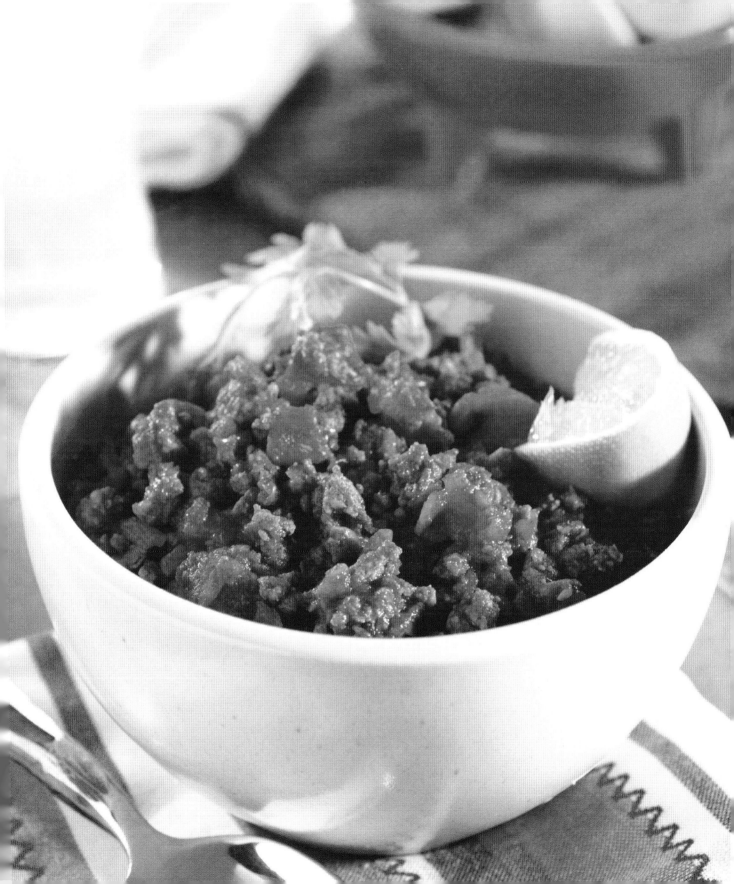

CHINESE PEPPERCORN BEEF

makes 4 servings

2 teaspoons whole black and pink peppercorns*

2 teaspoons coriander seeds

1 tablespoon peanut oil

1 boneless beef top sirloin steak, about 1¼ inches thick (1¼ pounds)

2 teaspoons dark sesame oil

½ cup thinly sliced shallots or sweet onion

½ cup chicken broth

2 tablespoons soy sauce

1 tablespoon dry sherry

2 tablespoons thinly sliced green onion or chopped fresh cilantro

Or use all black peppercorns if preferred.

1 Combine peppercorns and coriander seeds in small resealable food storage bag; seal bag. Coarsely crush spices with meat mallet or bottom of heavy saucepan. Brush peanut oil over both sides of steak; sprinkle with peppercorn mixture, pressing lightly to adhere.

2 Heat large heavy skillet over medium-high heat. Add steak; cook 4 minutes without moving or until seared on bottom. Reduce heat to medium; turn steak and cook 3 to 4 minutes for medium rare or until desired doneness. Remove steak to cutting board; tent with foil.

3 Add sesame oil to same skillet; heat over medium heat. Add shallots; cook 3 minutes, stirring frequently. Stir in broth, soy sauce and sherry; cook 5 minutes. Cut steak crosswise into thin slices. Spoon sauce over steak; sprinkle with green onion.

PER SERVING:

calories 330, *total fat* 14g, *carbs* 4g, *net carbs* 3g, *dietary fiber* 1g, *protein* 43g

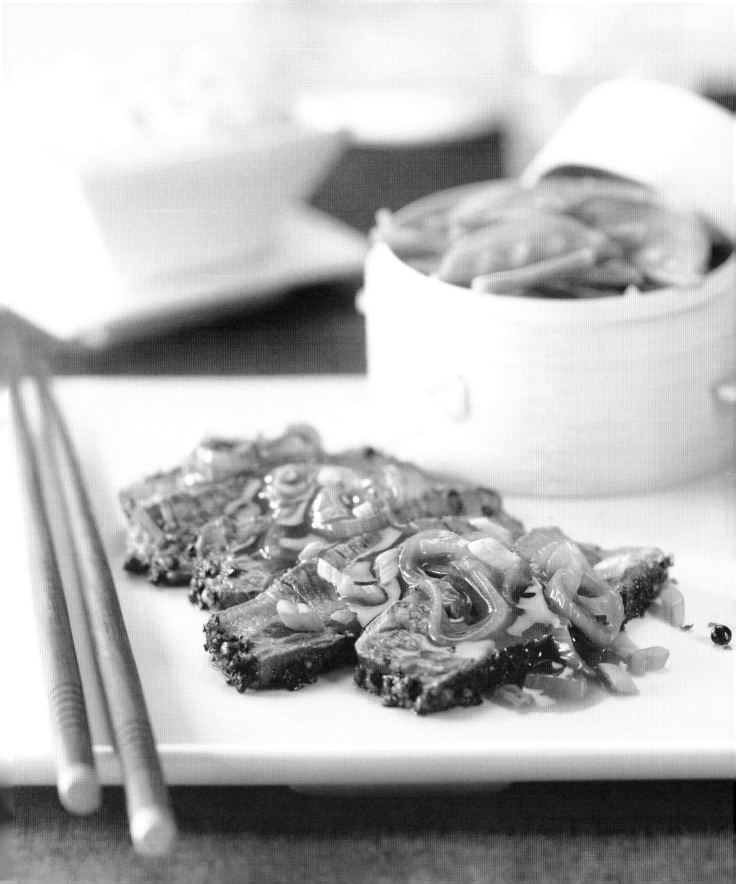

SAUSAGE AND PEPPERS

makes 4 servings

1 pound uncooked hot or mild Italian sausage links

2 tablespoons olive oil

3 medium onions, cut into ½-inch slices

2 red bell peppers, cut into ½-inch slices

2 green bell peppers, cut into ½-inch slices

1½ teaspoons coarse salt, divided

1 teaspoon dried oregano

1 Fill medium saucepan half full with water; bring to a boil over high heat. Add sausage; cook over medium heat 5 minutes. Drain sausage; cut diagonally into 1-inch slices.

2 Heat oil in large (12-inch) cast iron skillet over medium-high heat. Add sausage; cook about 10 minutes or until browned, stirring occasionally. Remove sausage to plate; set aside.

3 Add onions, bell peppers, 1 teaspoon salt and oregano to skillet; cook over medium heat about 25 minutes or until vegetables are very soft and browned in spots, stirring occasionally.

4 Stir sausage and remaining ½ teaspoon salt into skillet; cook 3 minutes or until heated through.

PER SERVING:

calories 510, *total fat* 43g, *carbs* 15g, *net carbs* 11g, *dietary fiber* 4g, *protein* 18g

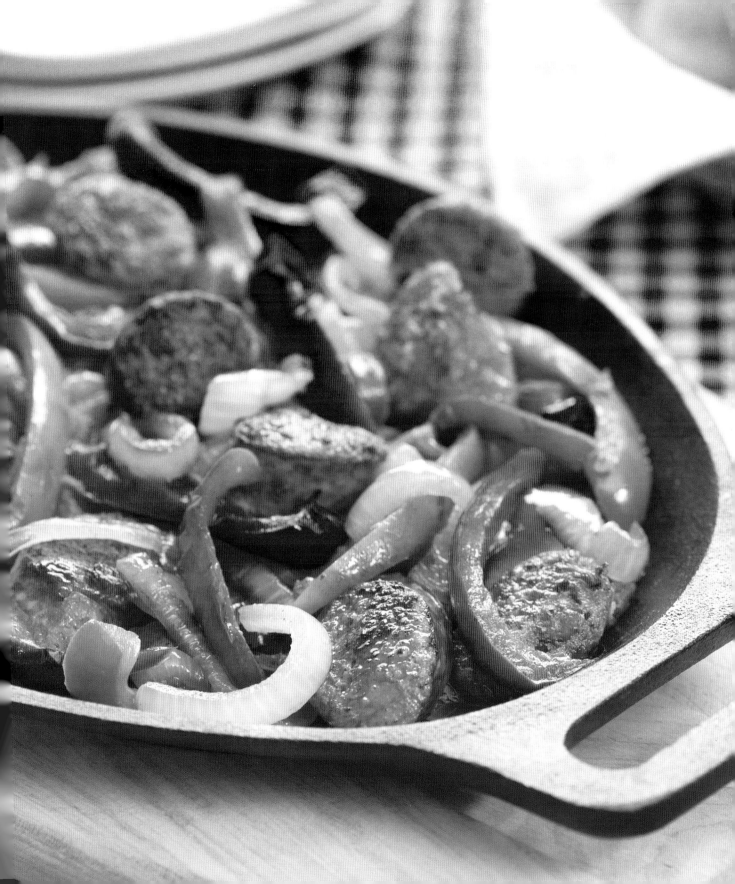

STEAK PARMESAN

makes 2 to 3 servings

4 cloves garlic, minced

1 tablespoon olive oil

1 tablespoon coarse salt

1 teaspoon black pepper

2 beef T-bone or Porterhouse steaks, 1 to 1¼ inches thick (about 2 pounds)

¼ cup grated Parmesan cheese

1 Prepare grill for direct cooking. Combine garlic, oil, salt and pepper in small bowl; mix well. Brush mixture on both sides of steaks; let stand 15 minutes.

2 Grill steaks, covered, over medium-high heat 14 to 19 minutes or until 145°F for medium rare, turning once.

3 Remove steaks to cutting board; sprinkle with cheese. Tent with foil; let stand 5 minutes before serving.

TIP: For a smoky flavor, soak 2 cups hickory or oak wood chips in cold water to cover at least 30 minutes. Drain and scatter over hot coals before grilling.

PER SERVING:

calories 855, *total fat* 57g, *carbs* 3g, *net carbs* 3g, *dietary fiber* 0g, *protein* 77g

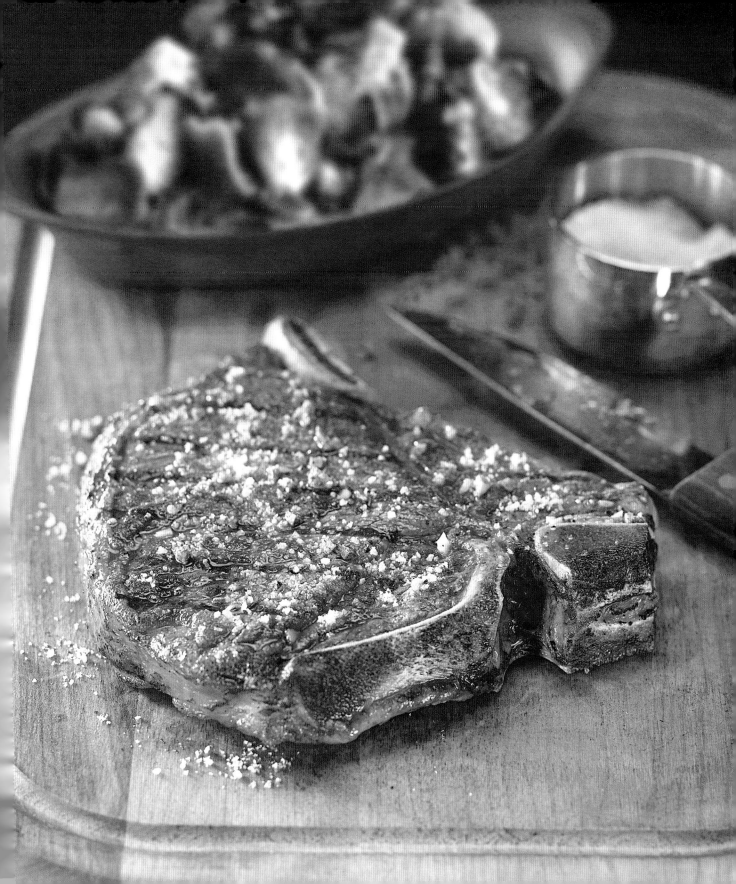

PORK TENDERLOIN
WITH CABBAGE AND LEEKS

makes 4 servings

¼ cup olive oil, plus additional for pan

1 teaspoon salt

¾ teaspoon garlic powder

½ teaspoon dried thyme

½ teaspoon black pepper

1 pork tenderloin (about 1¼ pounds)

½ medium savoy cabbage, cored and cut into ¼-inch slices (about 6 cups)

1 small leek, cut in half lengthwise then cut crosswise into ¼-inch diagonal slices

1 to 2 teaspoons cider vinegar

1 Preheat oven to 450°F. Brush baking sheet with oil.

2 Combine salt, garlic powder, thyme and pepper in small bowl; mix well. Stir in ¼ cup oil until well blended. Brush pork with about 1 tablespoon oil mixture, turning to coat all sides.

3 Combine cabbage and leek in large bowl. Drizzle with remaining oil mixture; toss to coat. Spread on prepared baking sheet; top with pork.

4 Roast about 25 minutes or until pork is 145°F, stirring cabbage mixture halfway through cooking time. Remove pork to cutting board; tent with foil. Let stand 10 minutes before slicing. Add vinegar to cabbage mixture; stir to blend.

TIP: If you can't find savoy cabbage, you can substitute regular green cabbage but it may take slightly longer to cook. If the cabbage is not crisp-tender when the pork is done, return the vegetables to the oven for 10 minutes or until crisp-tender.

PER SERVING:

calories 320, *total fat* 17g, *carbs* 10g, *net carbs* 6g, *dietary fiber* 4g, *protein* 32g

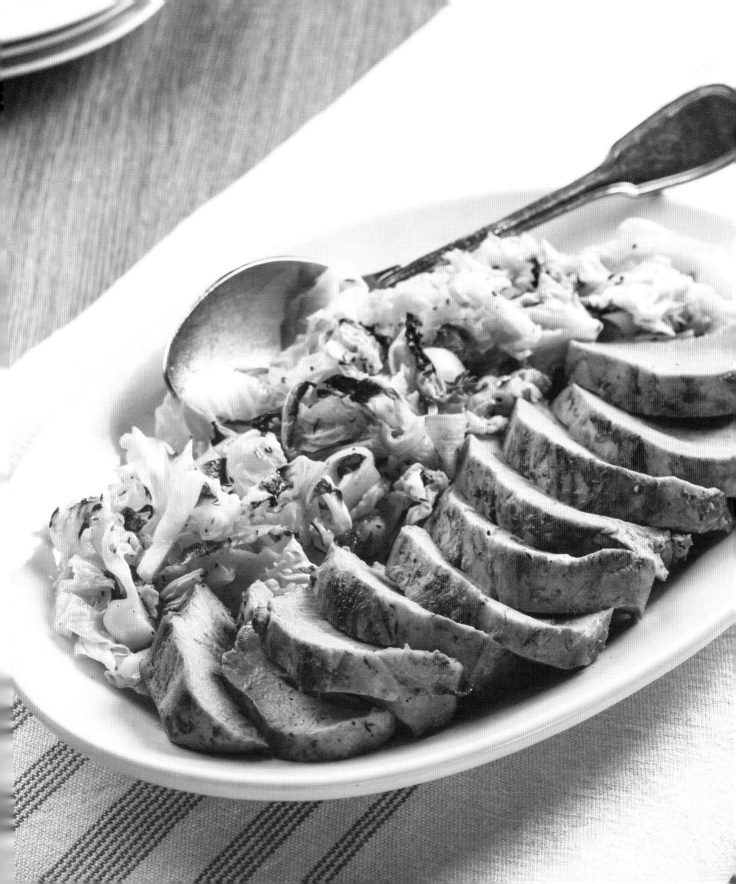

BEEF AND PEPPER KABOBS

makes 4 servings

8 ounces sirloin steak

2 teaspoons red wine vinegar

2 teaspoons reduced-sodium soy sauce

1½ teaspoons Dijon mustard

1 teaspoon olive oil

1 clove garlic, minced

⅛ teaspoon black pepper

2 small bell peppers (green, red, yellow and/or orange)

4 large green onions

1 tablespoon chicken or vegetable broth

1 Cut steak into 16 (¼-inch) strips; place in medium bowl. Whisk vinegar, soy sauce, mustard, oil, garlic and black pepper in small bowl until well blended. Add half of mixture to beef; stir to coat. Cover and refrigerate 2 to 3 hours, stirring occasionally. Cover remaining marinade and refrigerate until ready to grill.

2 Prepare grill for direct cooking. If using wooden skewers, soak in water 20 to 25 minutes before using to prevent burning. Cut each bell pepper into 12 pieces; thread onto four skewers.

3 Grill 5 to 7 minutes per side or until tender and well browned. Grill green onions 3 to 5 minutes or until well browned on both sides. Stir broth into reserved marinade; brush lightly over bell peppers and green onions once during grilling.

4 Thread 4 beef strips onto each of four skewers. Grill 2 minutes per side, basting each side once with marinade. Coarsely chop green onions; sprinkle over skewers.

PER SERVING:

calories 105, *total fat* 4g, *carbs* 4g, *net carbs* 3g, *dietary fiber* 1g, *protein* 14g

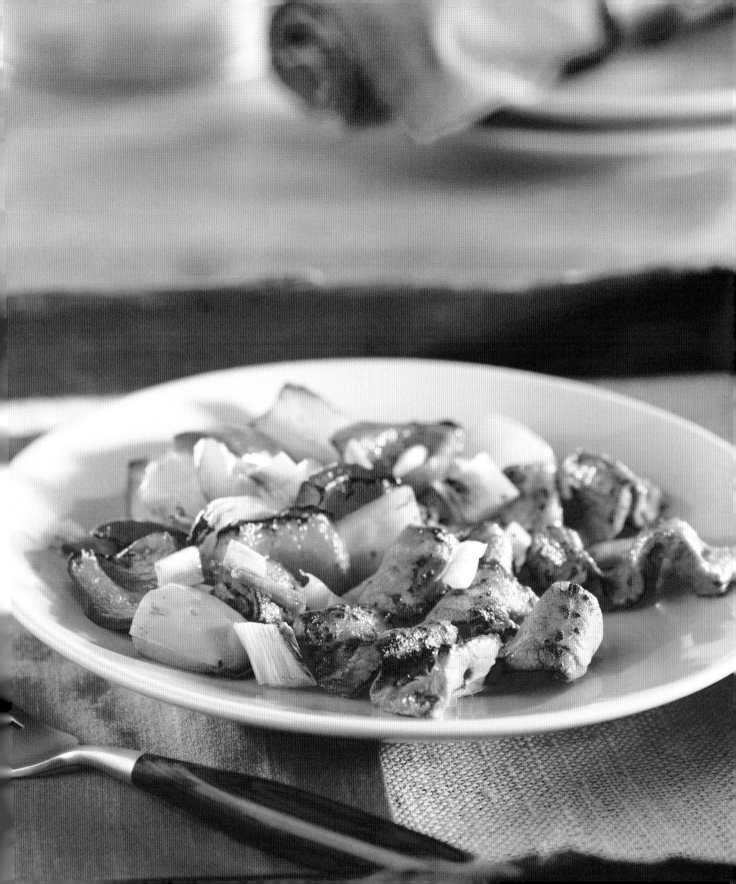

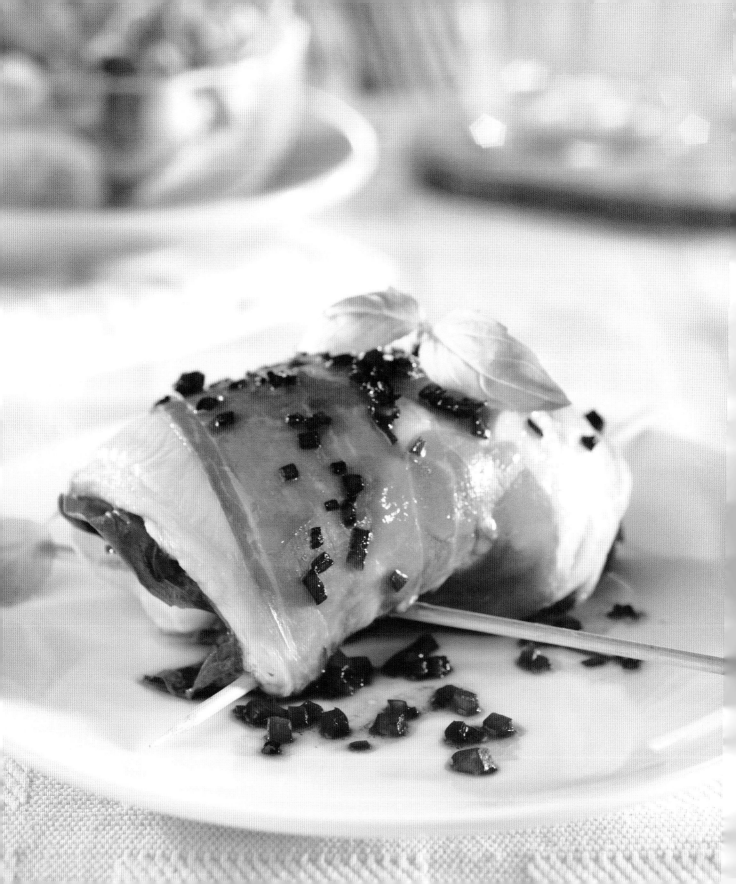

POULTRY

PROSCIUTTO-WRAPPED CHICKEN WITH GOAT CHEESE

makes 4 servings

8 slices lean prosciutto

4 boneless skinless chicken breasts (4 ounces each)

2 to 3 ounces goat cheese

16 to 24 basil leaves, plus additional for garnish

1 teaspoon olive oil

1 shallot, finely chopped

2 tablespoons dry red wine

1 Preheat oven to 350°F. Spray 8- or 9-inch baking dish with nonstick cooking spray.

2 Pound chicken to ¼-inch thickness between sheets of waxed paper or plastic wrap with flat side of meat mallet or rolling pin. Cut each chicken breast in half crosswise.

3 Lay prosciutto slices on clean work surface or cutting board. Place 1 piece chicken on top of each piece of prosciutto. Top with cheese; arrange 2 to 3 basil leaves over cheese. Wrap prosciutto around chicken; secure with toothpicks. Place chicken in prepared baking dish.

4 Heat oil in small skillet over medium heat. Add shallot; cook and stir about 2 minutes or until softened. Add wine; cook and stir 1 minute. Pour mixture over chicken.

5 Bake 20 minutes. Garnish with additional basil.

PER SERVING:

calories 219, *total fat* 8g, *carbs* 1g, *net carbs* 1g, *dietary fiber* 0g, *protein* 31g

CREAMY BAKED CHICKEN WITH ARTICHOKES AND MUSHROOMS

makes 6 servings

6 boneless skinless chicken breasts (4 to 6 ounces each)

1½ teaspoons paprika

1½ teaspoons dried thyme

½ teaspoon salt

½ teaspoon black pepper

1 can (14 ounces) artichokes packed in water, drained

1 tablespoon butter

1 package (8 ounces) sliced cremini mushrooms

2 tablespoons almond flour

¾ cup reduced-sodium chicken broth

½ cup half-and-half

1 Preheat oven to 375°F.

2 Place chicken in 13×9-inch baking dish. Combine paprika, thyme, salt and pepper in small bowl; mix well. Reserve 1 teaspoon seasoning mixture; set aside. Sprinkle remaining seasoning mixture over chicken. Cut artichokes in half; arrange around chicken.

3 Melt butter in large saucepan over medium heat. Add mushrooms and reserved 1 teaspoon seasoning mixture; cook and stir 5 minutes or until tender. Sprinkle almond flour over mushrooms; cook and stir 1 minute. Stir in broth; cook 3 minutes or until thickened. Stir in half-and-half; cook and stir 1 minute. Pour over chicken and artichokes.

4 Bake 30 minutes or until chicken is no longer pink.

PER SERVING:

calories 220, *total fat* 6g, *carbs* 14g, *net carbs* 7g, *dietary fiber* 7g, *protein* 29g

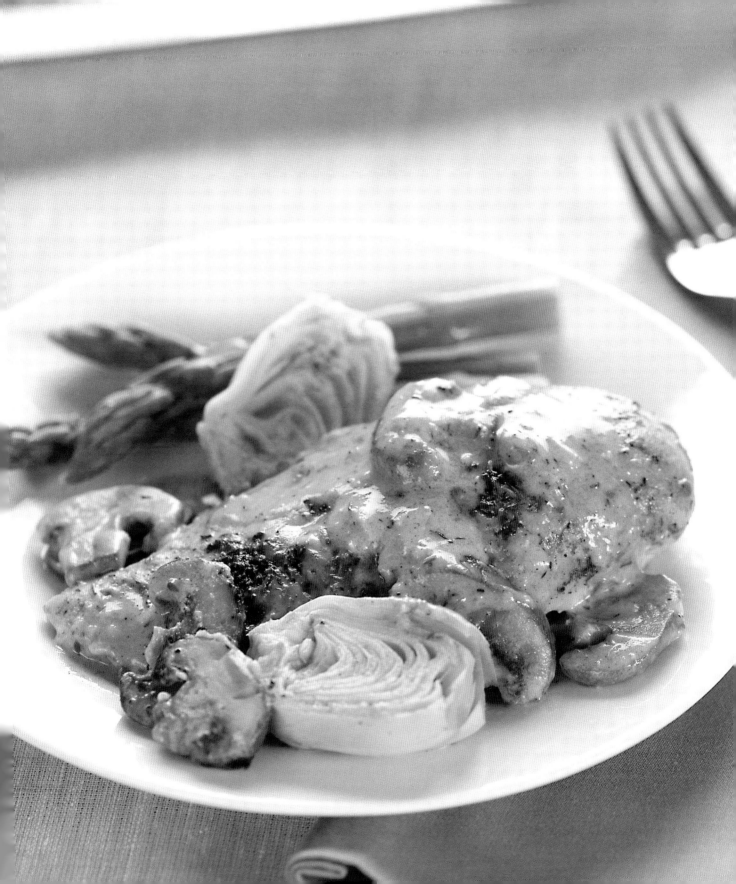

ROASTED TURKEY BREAST WITH SPINACH-BLUE CHEESE STUFFING

makes 7 servings

1 frozen whole boneless turkey breast (3½ to 4 pounds), thawed

1 package (10 ounces) frozen chopped spinach, thawed and squeezed dry

2 ounces blue cheese or feta cheese

2 ounces reduced-fat cream cheese (Neufchâtel), softened

½ cup finely chopped green onions

1½ tablespoons Dijon mustard

1½ tablespoons dried basil

2 teaspoons dried oregano

Salt, black pepper and paprika

1 Preheat oven to 350°F. Spray small roasting pan and rack with nonstick cooking spray.

2 Unroll turkey breast; pat dry. Pound turkey to 1-inch thickness between sheets of plastic wrap or waxed paper with flat side of meat mallet or rolling pin. Remove and discard skin from one half of turkey breast; turn meat over so skin side (on other half) faces down.

3 Combine spinach, blue cheese, cream cheese, green onions, mustard, basil and oregano in medium bowl; mix well. Spread evenly over turkey breast. Roll up turkey so skin is on top; tie closed with kitchen string. Place turkey on prepared rack; season with salt, pepper and paprika.

4 Roast 1½ hours or until no longer pink in center. Remove to cutting board; tent loosely with foil. Let stand 10 minutes. Remove skin; cut into into ¼-inch-thick slices.

PER SERVING:

calories 270, **total fat** 8g, **carbs** 4g, **net carbs** 2g, **dietary fiber** 2g, **protein** 44g

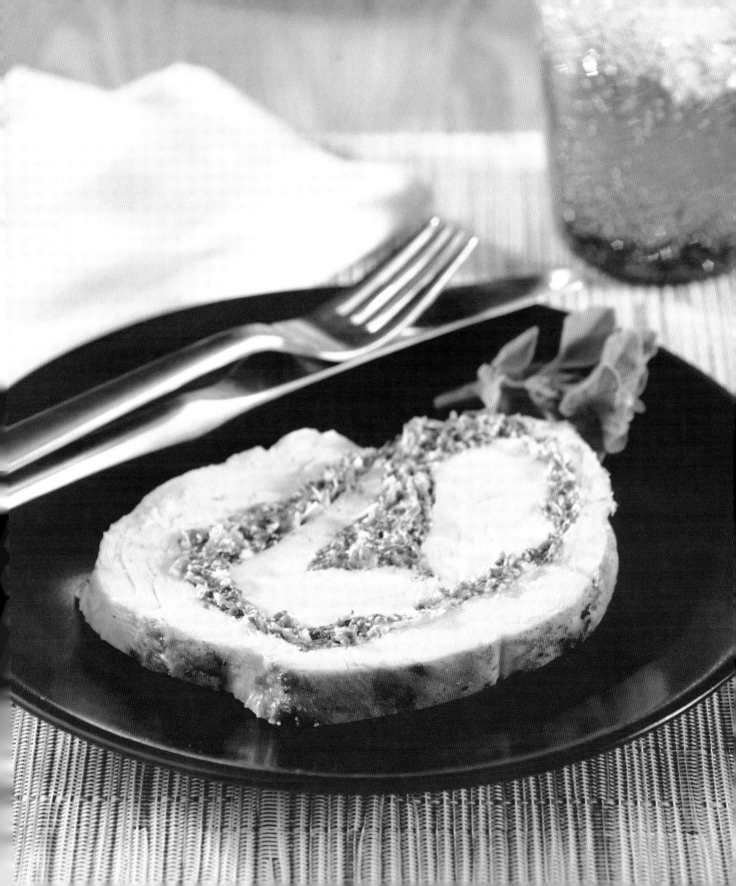

GREEK CHICKEN BURGERS WITH CUCUMBER YOGURT SAUCE

makes 4 servings

½ cup plus 2 tablespoons plain nonfat Greek yogurt

½ medium cucumber, peeled, seeded and finely chopped

Juice of ½ lemon

3 cloves garlic, minced, divided

2 teaspoons finely chopped fresh mint *or* ½ teaspoon dried mint

⅛ teaspoon salt

⅛ teaspoon ground white pepper

1 pound ground chicken breast

3 ounces reduced-fat crumbled feta cheese

4 large kalamata olives, rinsed, patted dry and minced

1 egg

½ teaspoon dried oregano

¼ teaspoon black pepper

Mixed greens (optional)

1 Combine yogurt, cucumber, lemon juice, 2 cloves garlic, mint, salt and white pepper in medium bowl; mix well. Cover and refrigerate until ready to serve.

2 Combine chicken, cheese, olives, egg, oregano, black pepper and remaining 1 clove garlic in large bowl; mix well. Shape mixture into four patties.

3 Spray grill pan with nonstick cooking spray; heat over medium-high heat. Grill patties 5 to 7 minutes per side or until cooked through (165°F).

4 Serve burgers with sauce and mixed greens, if desired.

PER SERVING:

calories 260, *total fat* 14g, *carbs* 4g, *net carbs* 3g, *dietary fiber* 1g, *protein* 29g

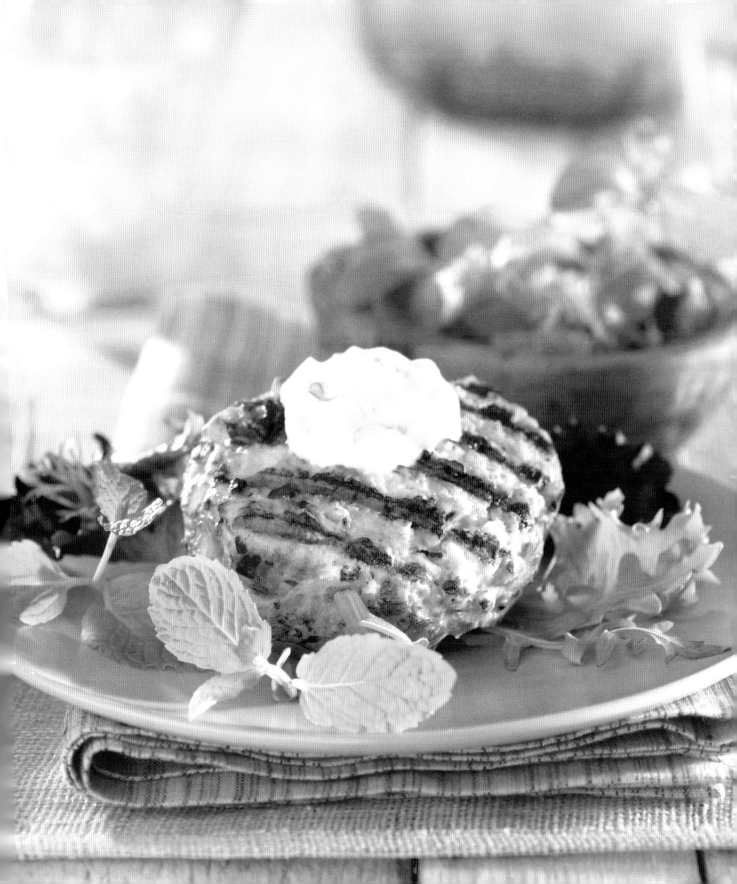

SHEET PAN CHICKEN
AND SAUSAGE SUPPER

makes 6 servings

⅓ cup olive oil

2 tablespoons balsamic vinegar

1 teaspoon salt

1 teaspoon garlic powder

½ teaspoon black pepper

¼ teaspoon red pepper flakes

3 pounds bone-in chicken thighs and drumsticks

1 pound uncooked sweet Italian sausage (4 to 5 links), cut diagonally into 2-inch pieces

6 small red onions (about 1 pound), each cut into 6 wedges

3½ cups broccoli florets

1 Preheat oven to 425°F. Line baking sheet with foil, if desired.

2 Whisk oil, vinegar, salt, garlic powder, black pepper and red pepper flakes in small bowl until well blended. Combine chicken, sausage and onions on prepared baking sheet. Drizzle with oil mixture; toss to coat. Spread meat and onions in single layer (chicken thighs should be skin side up).

3 Bake 30 minutes. Add broccoli to baking sheet; stir to coat broccoli with pan juices and turn sausage. Bake 30 minutes or until broccoli begins to brown and chicken is cooked through (165°F).

PER SERVING:

calories 430, *total fat* 25g, *carbs* 12g, *net carbs* 10g, *dietary fiber* 2g, *protein* 41g

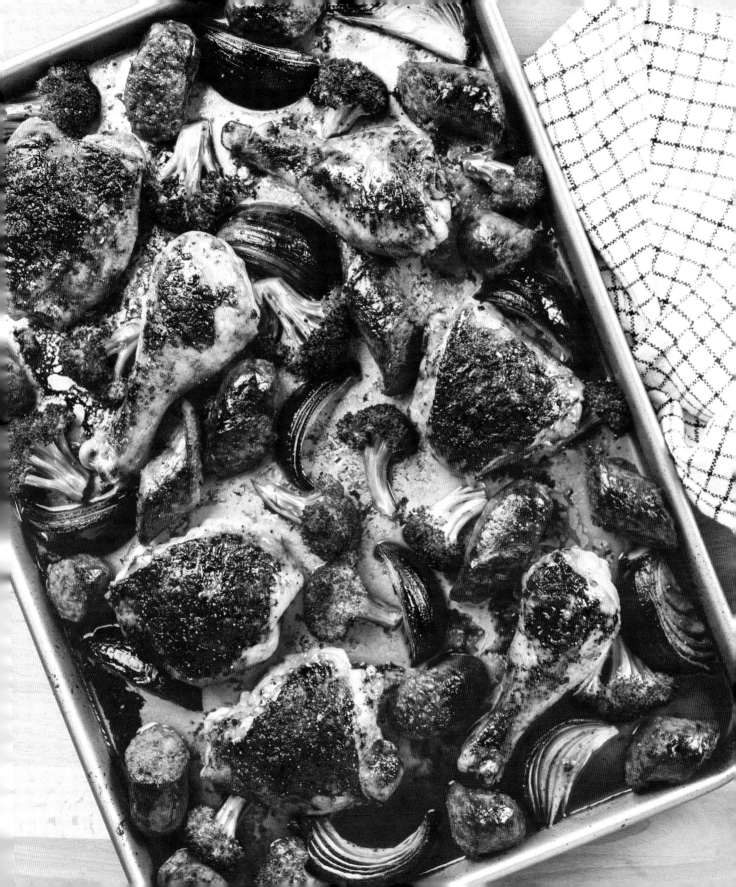

GRILLED CHICKEN ADOBO

makes 4 servings

½ cup chopped onion

⅓ cup lime juice

6 cloves garlic, coarsely chopped

1 teaspoon dried oregano

1 teaspoon ground cumin

½ teaspoon dried thyme

¼ teaspoon ground red pepper

4 boneless skinless chicken breasts (about 1 pound total)

2 tablespoons chopped fresh cilantro (optional)

1 Combine onion, lime juice and garlic in food processor; process until onion is finely minced. Transfer to large resealable food storage bag.

2 Add oregano, cumin, thyme and red pepper; knead bag until blended. Place chicken in bag; seal bag and turn to coat. Marinate in refrigerator 30 minutes or up to 4 hours, turning occasionally.

3 Prepare grill for direct cooking. Spray grid with nonstick cooking spray. Remove chicken from marinade; discard marinade.

4 Grill chicken over medium heat 5 to 7 minutes per side or until no longer pink in center. Garnish with cilantro.

PER SERVING:

calories 139, *total fat* 3g, *carbs* 1g, *net carbs* 0g, *dietary fiber* 1g, *protein* 25g

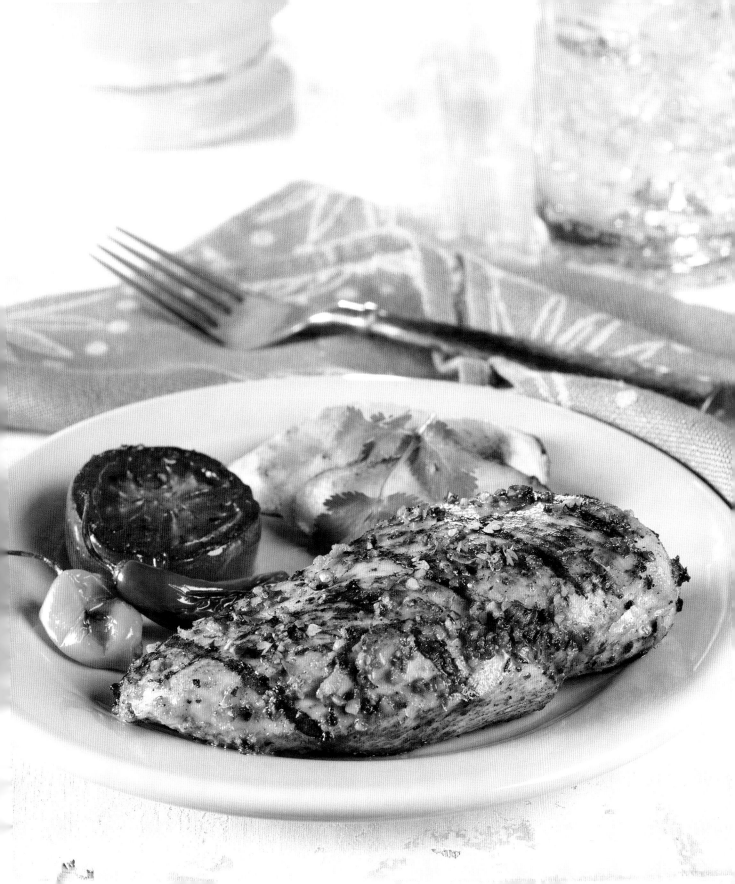

HERB ROASTED CHICKEN

makes 4 servings

1 whole chicken (3 to 4 pounds)	4 sprigs fresh rosemary, divided
1¼ teaspoons salt, divided	4 sprigs fresh thyme, divided
½ teaspoon black pepper, divided	4 cloves garlic, peeled
1 lemon, cut into quarters	2 tablespoons olive oil

1 Preheat oven to 425°F. Place chicken, breast side up, in shallow roasting pan. Season cavity of chicken with ½ teaspoon salt and ¼ teaspoon pepper. Fill cavity with lemon quarters, 2 sprigs rosemary, 2 sprigs thyme and garlic cloves.

2 Chop remaining rosemary and thyme leaves; combine with oil, remaining ¾ teaspoon salt and ¼ teaspoon pepper in small bowl. Brush mixture over chicken.

3 Roast 30 minutes. *Reduce oven temperature to 375°F;* roast 35 to 45 minutes or until cooked through (165°F). Remove to cutting board; tent with foil. Let stand 10 to 15 minutes before carving.

PER SERVING:

calories 280, *total fat* 15g, *carbs* 4g, *net carbs* 3g, *dietary fiber* 1g, *protein* 32g

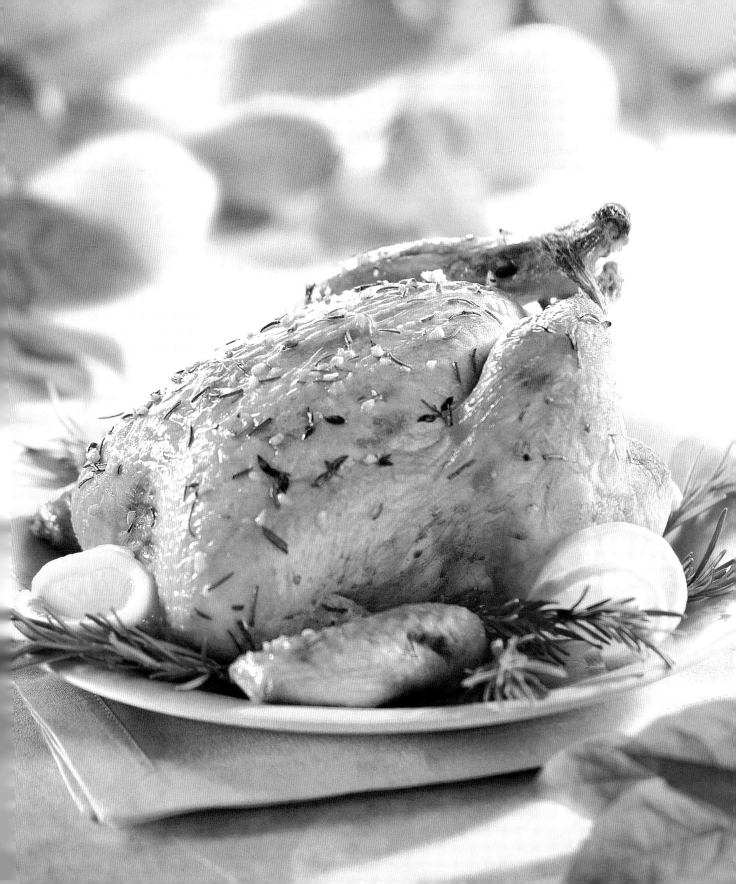

DUCK BREASTS WITH BALSAMIC SAUCE

makes 4 servings

3 tablespoons balsamic vinegar

2 tablespoons lemon juice

4 boneless duck breasts (6 ounces each)

Salt and black pepper

1 shallot, minced

1 Combine vinegar and lemon juice in small bowl; mix well.

2 Score skin on duck breasts with tip of sharp knife in crosshatch pattern, being careful to cut only into fat layer and not into meat. Season both sides of duck with salt and pepper.

3 Place duck breasts skin side down in large skillet over medium heat; cook without turning 10 to 12 minutes or until skin is crisp and golden brown. Turn and cook about 8 minutes or until medium rare (130°F). Remove duck to plate; tent with foil. Let stand 10 minutes before slicing.

4 Meanwhile, drain all but 1 tablespoon fat from skillet. Add shallot to skillet; cook and stir over medium heat 2 to 3 minutes or until translucent. Add vinegar mixture; cook and stir about 5 minutes or until slightly thickened. Season with salt and pepper. Slice duck; drizzle with sauce.

PER SERVING:

calories 360, *total fat* 18g, *carbs* 5g, *net carbs* 5g, *dietary fiber* 0g, *protein* 42g

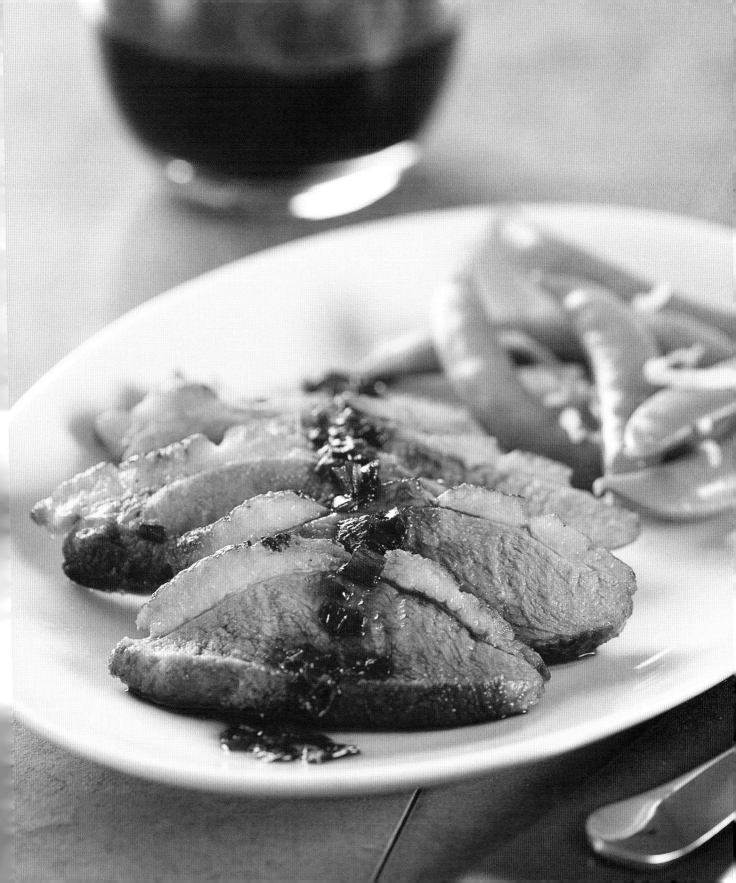

ROASTED CHICKEN WITH CABBAGE

makes 4 servings

⅓ cup olive oil, plus additional for pan

2 tablespoons red wine vinegar

2 cloves garlic, minced

1 teaspoon salt

1 teaspoon onion powder

¼ teaspoon paprika

¼ teaspoon black pepper

1½ medium onions, cut into ½-inch slices (do not separate into rings)

1 small head green cabbage (about 1½ pounds)

8 bone-in, skin-on chicken thighs (about 3 pounds)

Chopped fresh parsley (optional)

1 Preheat oven to 425°F. Brush baking sheet with oil.

2 Whisk ⅓ cup oil, vinegar, garlic, salt, onion powder, paprika and pepper in small bowl until well blended. Place onions in large bowl; drizzle with 2 tablespoons oil mixture and turn to coat. Arrange in single layer on prepared baking sheet.

3 Cut cabbage in half through core (do not remove core). Cut each half into 1-inch wedges Add cabbage to same bowl; drizzle with 2 tablespoons oil mixture and turn to coat. Arrange cabbage over onions on baking sheet. Add chicken to bowl; drizzle with remaining oil mixture and turn to coat. Place chicken, skin side up, over cabbage.

4 Roast 50 to 55 minutes or until chicken is 165°F. Remove chicken to plate; tent with foil. Carefully drain liquid from baking sheet. Stir vegetables; roast 10 to 15 minutes or until edges begin to brown and cabbage is crisp-tender. Serve chicken with vegetables. Garnish with parsley.

PER SERVING:

calories 480, **total fat** 27g, *carbs* 15g, **net carbs** 10g, **dietary fiber** 5g, **protein** 43g

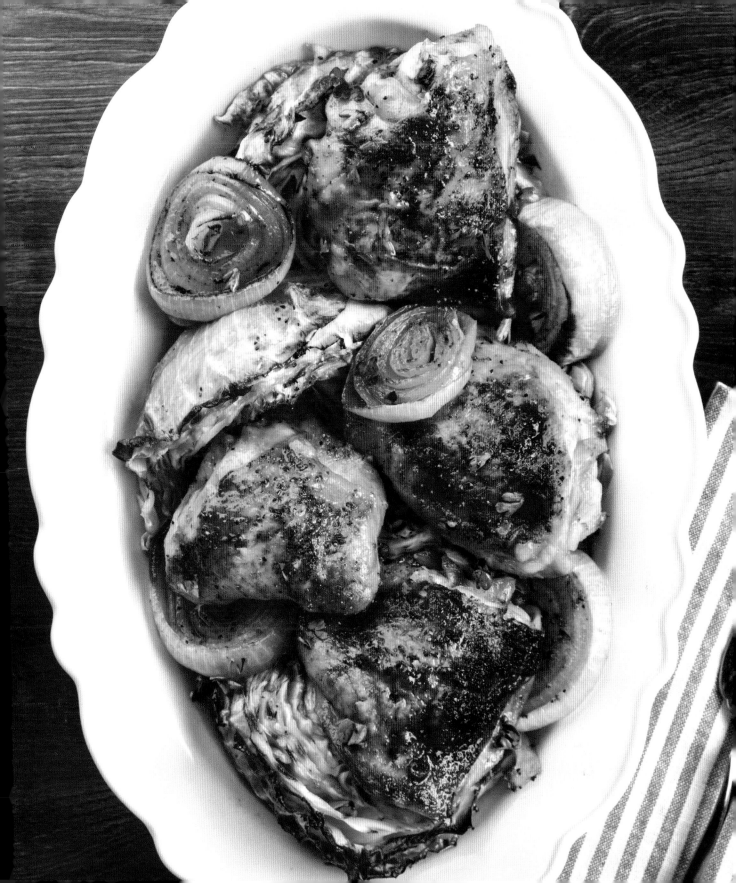

CHEESY CHICKEN WITH BACON AND MUSHROOMS

makes 4 servings

½ cup Dijon mustard

4 tablespoons olive oil, divided

1 teaspoon lemon juice

4 boneless skinless chicken breasts (about 6 ounces each)

Salt and black pepper

1 tablespoon butter

2 cups sliced mushrooms

4 slices bacon, cooked

½ cup (2 ounces) shredded Cheddar cheese

½ cup (2 ounces) shredded Monterey Jack cheese

Chopped fresh parsley

1 Whisk mustard, 3 tablespoons oil and lemon juice in medium bowl until well blended. Remove half of marinade mixture to use as sauce; cover and refrigerate until ready to serve.

2 Place chicken in large resealable food storage bag. Pour remaining half of marinade over chicken; seal bag and turn to coat. Marinate in refrigerator at least 2 hours.

3 Preheat oven to 375°F. Remove chicken from marinade; discard marinade. Heat remaining 1 tablespoon oil in large ovenproof skillet over medium-high heat. Add chicken; cook 3 to 4 minutes per side or until golden brown. (Chicken will not be cooked through.) Remove chicken to plate; sprinkle with salt and pepper.

4 Heat butter in same skillet over medium-high heat. Add mushrooms; cook 8 minutes or until mushrooms begin to brown, stirring occasionally and scraping up browned bits from bottom of skillet. Season with salt and pepper. Return chicken to skillet; spoon mushrooms over chicken. Top with bacon; sprinkle with Cheddar and Monterey Jack.

5 Bake 8 to 10 minutes or until chicken is no longer pink in center and cheeses are melted. Sprinkle with parsley; serve with reserved mustard mixture.

PER SERVING:

calories 610, *total fat* 41g, *carbs* 2g, *net carbs* 2g, *dietary fiber* 0g, *protein* 49g

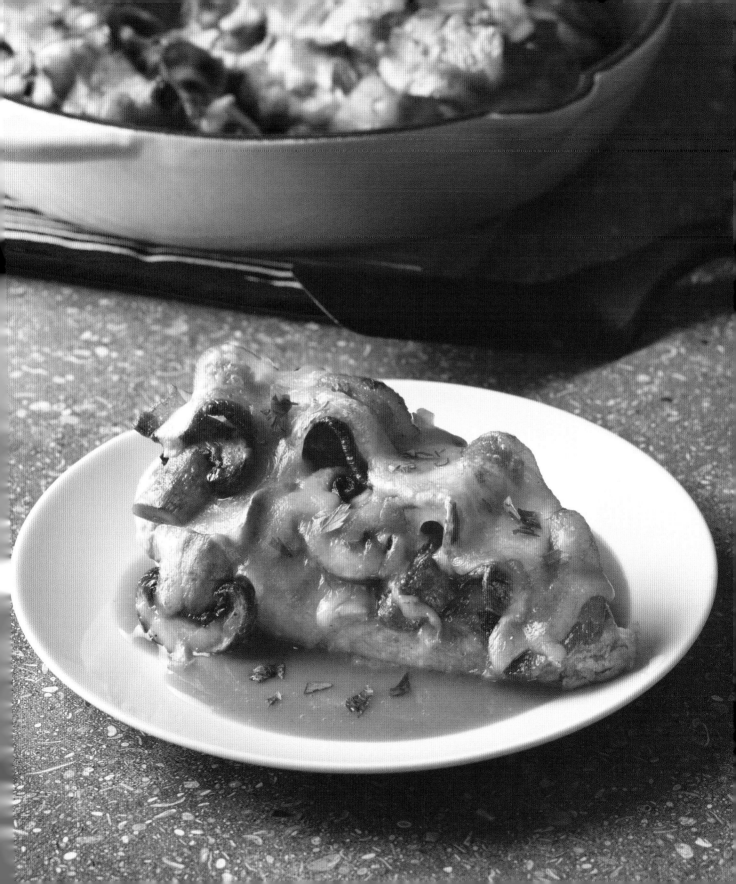

SPICED TARRAGON
ROASTED TURKEY BREAST

makes 6 servings

2 tablespoons safflower oil

2 teaspoons grated orange peel

1½ teaspoons dried tarragon

1 teaspoon ground cumin

½ teaspoon salt

½ teaspoon ground ginger

½ teaspoon ground allspice

½ teaspoon ground cinnamon

½ teaspoon black pepper

¼ teaspoon ground red pepper

1 frozen bone-in turkey breast half (2½ to 3 pounds), thawed

1 Preheat oven to 400°F. Whisk oil, orange peel, tarragon, cumin, salt, ginger, allspice, cinnamon, black pepper and red pepper in small bowl until well blended. Loosen skin from turkey; gently rub spice mixture under skin.

2 Spray small roasting pan with nonstick cooking spray. Place turkey, skin side up, in prepared pan.

3 Roast 1 hour 15 minutes or until cooked through (165°F). Remove to cutting board; tent with foil. Let stand 15 minutes before slicing. Remove and discard skin, leaving spice mixture on turkey. Cut into thin slices.

PER SERVING:

calories 220, *total fat* 7g, *carbs* 1g, *net carbs* 1g, *dietary fiber* 0g, *protein* 36g

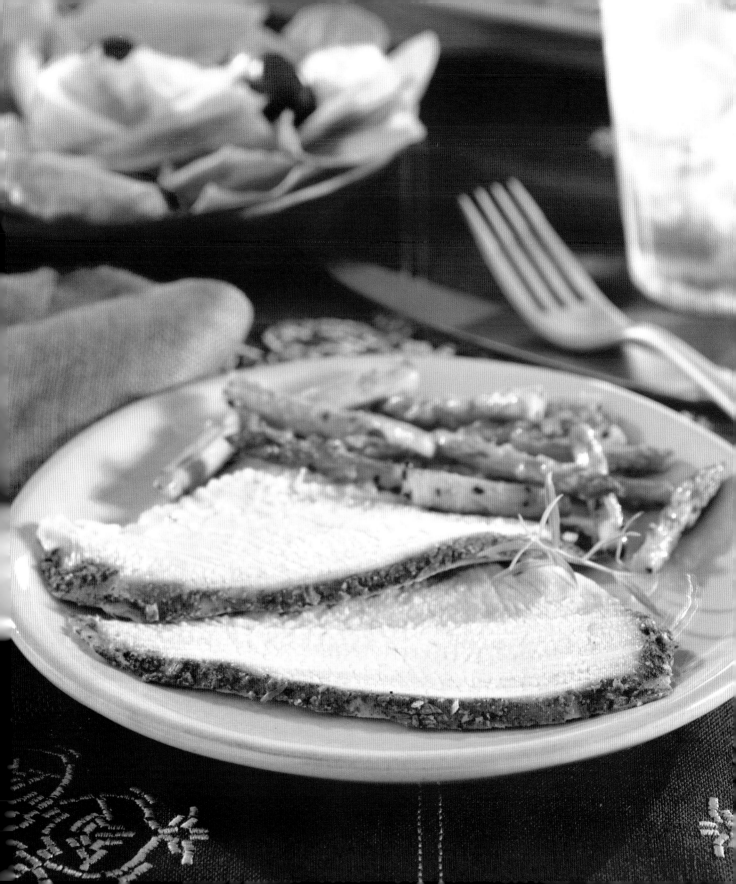

GARLICKY GREEK CHICKEN

makes 4 servings

12 cloves garlic, unpeeled

3 pounds chicken thighs and drumsticks

4 tablespoons lemon juice, divided

3 tablespoons olive oil

2 tablespoons chopped fresh rosemary leaves *or* 2 teaspoons dried rosemary

¾ teaspoon salt

½ teaspoon black pepper

1 teaspoon grated lemon peel

Additional fresh rosemary sprigs and lemon wedges for garnish

1 Preheat oven to 375°F. Place garlic in shallow roasting pan; arrange chicken over garlic. Whisk 2 tablespoons lemon juice, oil and chopped rosemary in small bowl until well blended. Spoon evenly over chicken; sprinkle with salt and pepper.

2 Bake 50 to 55 minutes or until chicken is cooked through (165°F). Remove to platter; tent with foil.

3 Squeeze garlic pulp from skins; discard skins. Place garlic pulp in roasting pan; add remaining 2 tablespoons lemon juice. Cook over medium heat, mashing garlic and scraping up browned bits from bottom of pan.

4 Pour sauce over chicken; sprinkle with lemon peel. Garnish with rosemary sprigs and lemon wedges.

TIP: Unpeeled cloves of garlic usually burst open while roasting, making it a cinch to squeeze out the softened, creamy roasted garlic with your thumb and forefinger. If the cloves have not burst open, simply cut off the end with a knife and squeeze out the garlic.

PER SERVING:

calories 592, **total fat** 43g, *carbs* 5g, **net carbs** 4g, *dietary fiber* 1g, *protein* 45g

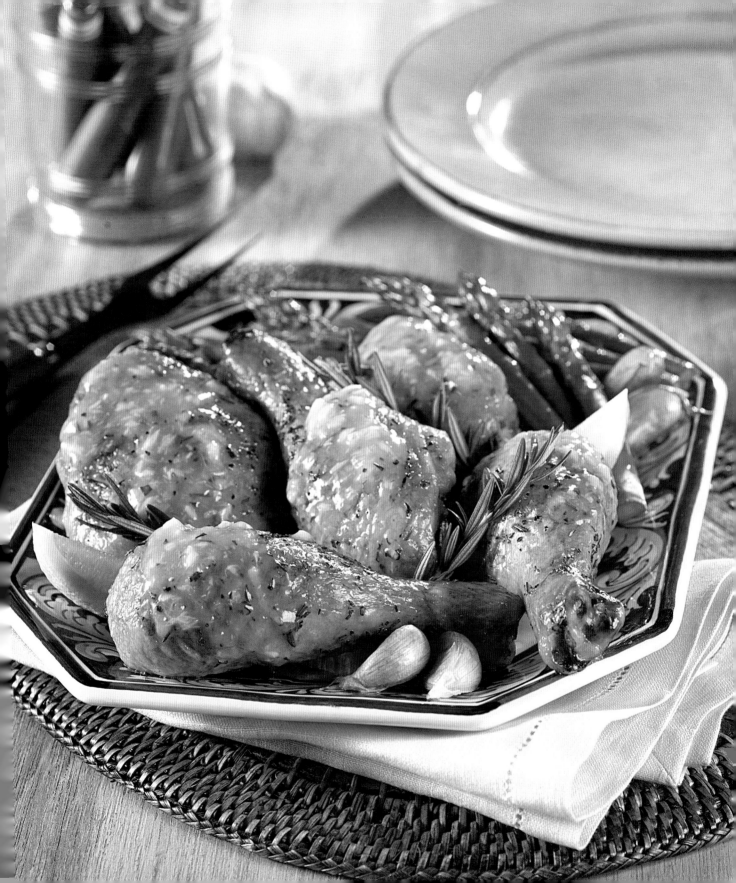

KALE AND MUSHROOM
STUFFED CHICKEN BREASTS

makes 4 servings

3 teaspoons olive oil, divided

1 cup coarsely chopped mushrooms

2 cups thinly sliced kale

1 tablespoon fresh lemon juice

½ teaspoon salt, divided

4 boneless skinless chicken breasts (about 4 ounces each)

¼ cup crumbled fat-free feta cheese

¼ teaspoon black pepper

1 Heat 1 teaspoon oil in large skillet over medium-high heat. Add mushrooms; cook and stir 5 minutes or until mushrooms begin to brown. Add kale; cook and stir 8 minutes or until wilted. Sprinkle with lemon juice and ¼ teaspoon salt. Remove to small bowl; let stand 5 to 10 minutes to cool slightly.

2 Meanwhile, pound chicken to ½-inch thickness between sheets of waxed paper or plastic wrap with flat side of meat mallet or rolling pin.

3 Gently stir cheese into mushroom mixture. Spoon ¼ cup mixture down center of each chicken breast. Roll up to enclose filling; secure with toothpicks. Sprinkle with remaining ¼ teaspoon salt and pepper.

4 Wipe out same skillet with paper towels. Add remaining 2 teaspoons oil to skillet; heat over medium heat. Add chicken; cook until browned on all sides. Cover and cook 5 minutes per side or until no longer pink. Remove toothpicks before serving.

PER SERVING:
calories 192, **total fat** 7g, **carbs** 4g, **net carbs** 3g, **dietary fiber** 1g, **protein** 29g

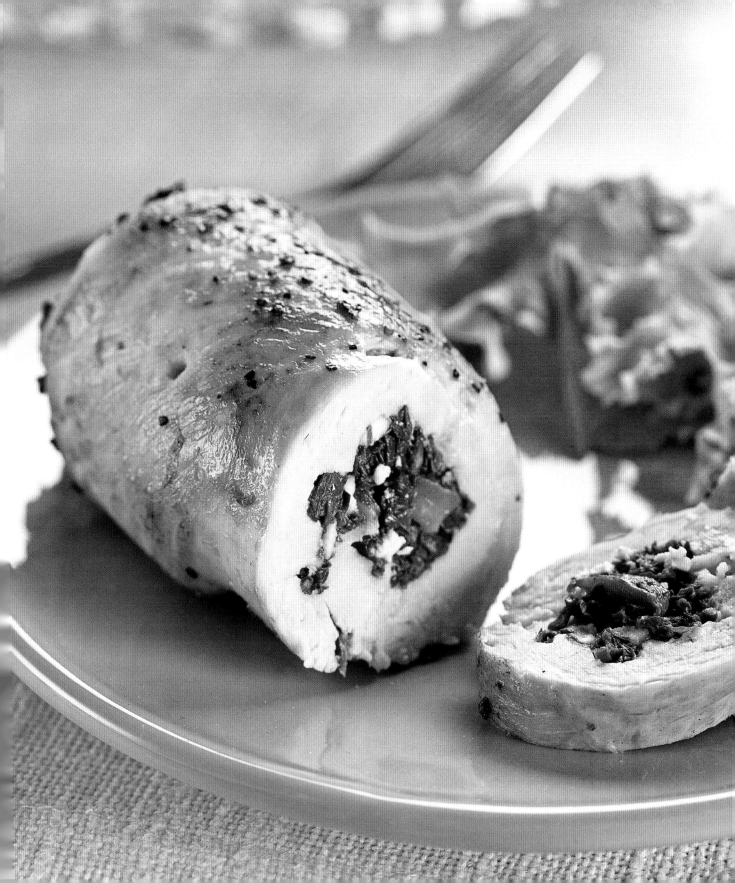

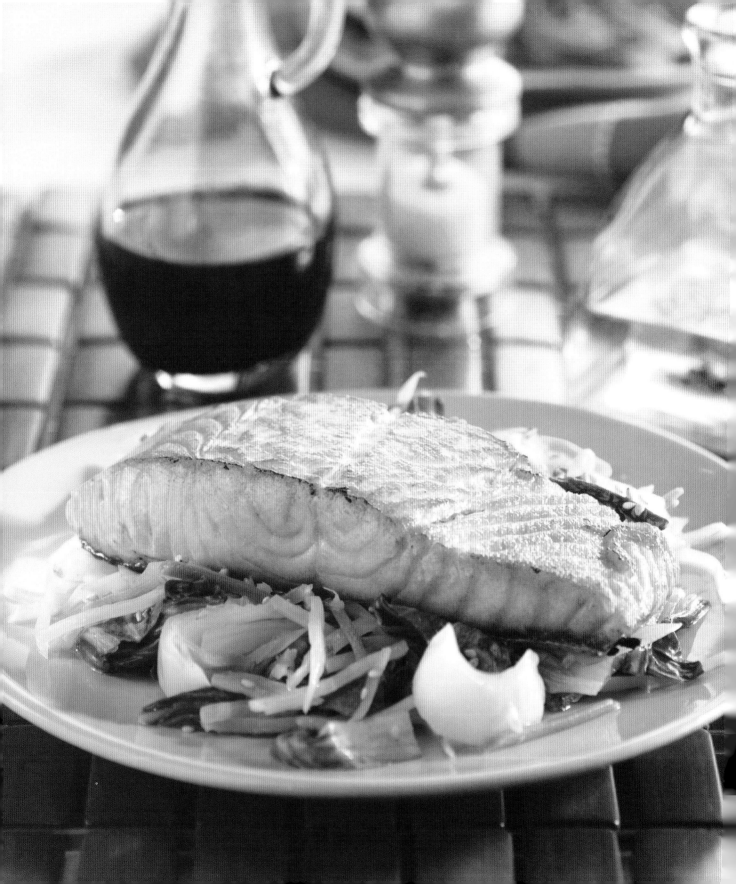

SEAFOOD

PAN-COOKED BOK CHOY SALMON

makes 2 servings

1 pound bok choy or napa cabbage, chopped

1 cup broccoli slaw mix

2 tablespoons olive oil, divided

2 salmon fillets (4 to 6 ounces each)

½ teaspoon black pepper

¼ teaspoon salt

1 teaspoon sesame seeds

1 Combine bok choy and broccoli slaw mix in colander; rinse and drain well.

2 Heat 1 tablespoon oil in large skillet over medium heat. Sprinkle salmon with ½ teaspoon pepper and ¼ teaspoon salt. Add to skillet; cook 3 minutes per side. Remove to plate.

3 Add remaining 1 tablespoon oil and sesame seeds to skillet; cook and stir 2 to 3 minutes or until seeds are golden brown. Add bok choy mixture; cook and stir 3 to 4 minutes.

4 Return fish to skillet. Reduce heat to low; cover and cook 4 minutes or until fish begins to flake when tested with fork. Season with additional salt and pepper, if desired.

PER SERVING:

calories 410, *total fat* 30g, *carbs* 8g, *net carbs* 5g, *dietary fiber* 3g, *protein* 28g

LEMON ROSEMARY SHRIMP AND VEGETABLE SOUVLAKI

makes 4 servings

8 ounces large raw shrimp, peeled and deveined (with tails on)

1 medium zucchini, halved lengthwise and cut into ½-inch slices

½ medium red bell pepper, cut into 1-inch pieces

8 green onions, trimmed and cut into 2-inch pieces

2 tablespoons extra virgin olive oil

2 tablespoons lemon juice

2 teaspoons grated lemon peel

2 medium cloves garlic, minced

½ teaspoon salt

½ teaspoon fresh rosemary

⅛ teaspoon red pepper flakes

1 Prepare grill for direct cooking. Spray grid or grill pan with nonstick cooking spray.

2 Spray four 12-inch bamboo or metal skewers with cooking spray. If using bamboo skewers, soak in water 20 to 30 minutes before using to prevent burning. Alternately thread shrimp, zucchini, bell pepper and green onions onto skewers. Spray skewers lightly with cooking spray.

3 Whisk oil, lemon juice, lemon peel, garlic, salt, rosemary and red pepper flakes in small bowl until well blended.

4 Grill skewers over high heat 2 minutes per side. Remove to platter; drizzle with sauce.

NOTE: "Souvlaki" is the Greek word for shishkebab. Souvlaki traditionally consists of fish or meat that has been seasoned in a mixture of oil, lemon juice, and seasonings. Many souvlaki recipes, including this one, also include chunks of vegetables such as bell pepper and onion.

PER SERVING:

calories 130, *total fat* 8g, *carbs* 6g, *net carbs* 4g, *dietary fiber* 2g, *protein* 9g

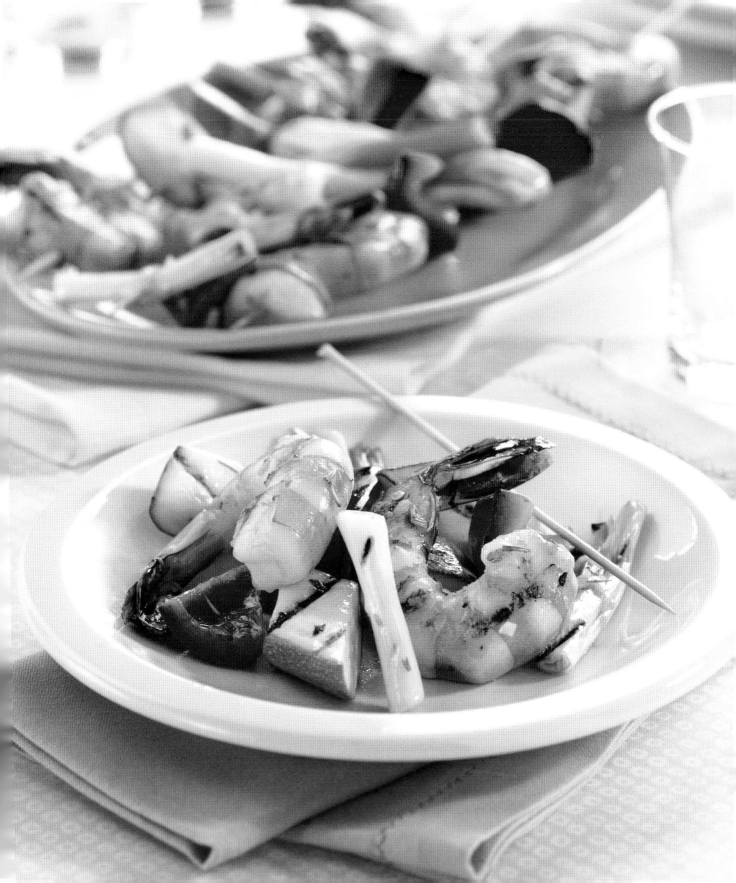

TUNA WITH SPICY HORSERADISH SAUCE

makes 4 servings

½ cup sour cream

1 tablespoon water

2 teaspoons prepared horseradish

1 teaspoon Dijon mustard

1 medium clove garlic, minced

½ teaspoon dried rosemary

½ teaspoon salt

4 fresh tuna steaks (4 ounces each), rinsed and patted dry

2 teaspoons steak seasoning blend

2 tablespoons finely chopped green onion or fresh parsley

1 Whisk sour cream, water, horseradish, mustard, garlic, rosemary and salt in small bowl until well blended.

2 Sprinkle both sides of tuna with steak seasoning blend, pressing to adhere.

3 Spray grill pan with nonstick cooking spray; heat over medium-high heat. Cook fish 1½ minutes per side. *Do not overcook or tuna will be tough and dry.* Sprinkle with green onion; serve with sauce.

PER SERVING:

calories 200, *total fat* 6g, *carbs* 3g, *net carbs* 3g, *dietary fiber* 0g, *protein* 29g

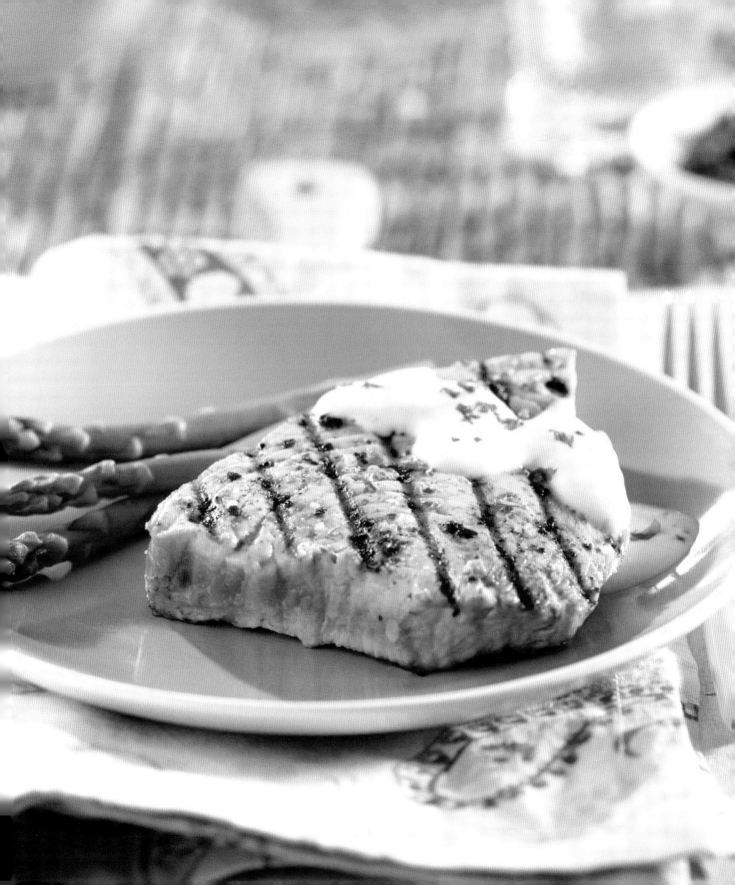

GRILLED TILAPIA WITH ZESTY MUSTARD SAUCE

makes 4 servings

1 tablespoon olive oil

1 teaspoon Dijon mustard

½ teaspoon grated lemon peel

½ teaspoon Worcestershire sauce

½ teaspoon salt, divided

¼ teaspoon black pepper

4 tilapia fillets (about 4 ounces each)

1½ teaspoons paprika

½ medium lemon, quartered

1 Prepare grill for direct cooking. Lightly spray grill basket with cooking spray.

2 Combine oil, mustard, lemon peel, Worcestershire sauce, ¼ teaspoon salt and pepper in small bowl; mix well.

3 Rinse tilapia; pat dry with paper towels. Sprinkle both sides of fish with paprika and remaining ¼ teaspoon salt. Place fish in prepared basket.

4 Grill, covered, over high heat 3 minutes. Turn and grill, covered, 2 to 3 minutes, or until fish begins to flake when tested with fork. Squeeze one lemon wedge over each fillet. Spread mustard mixture over fish.

PER SERVING:

calories 136, *total fat* 5g, *carbs* 1g, *net carbs* 0g, *dietary fiber* 1g, *protein* 23g

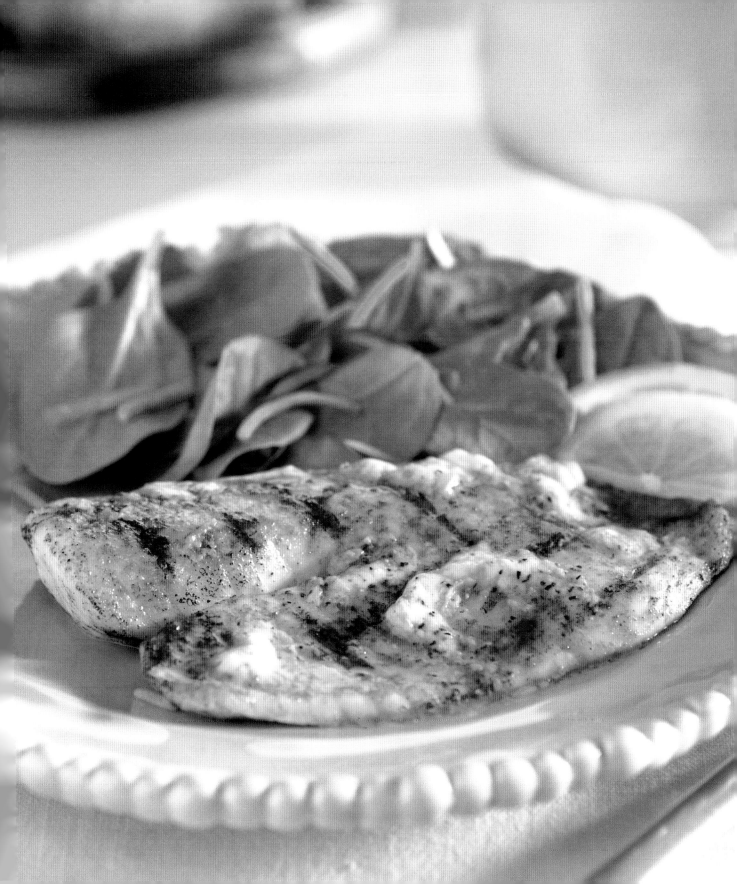

SHRIMP AND VEGGIE SKILLET

makes 4 servings

¼ cup reduced-sodium soy sauce

2 tablespoons lime juice

1 tablespoon sesame oil

1 teaspoon grated fresh ginger

⅛ teaspoon red pepper flakes

32 medium raw shrimp (about 8 ounces total), peeled and deveined (with tails on)

2 medium zucchini, cut in half lengthwise and thinly sliced

6 green onions, trimmed and halved lengthwise

12 grape tomatoes

1 Whisk soy sauce, lime juice, oil, ginger and red pepper flakes in small bowl until well blended.

2 Spray large nonstick skillet with nonstick cooking spray; heat over medium-high heat. Add shrimp; cook and stir 3 minutes or until shrimp are opaque. Remove to plate.

3 Spray same skillet with cooking spray. Add zucchini; cook and stir 4 to 6 minutes or just until crisp-tender. Add green onions and tomatoes; cook 1 to 2 minutes or until green onions begin to wilt. Add shrimp, cook 1 minute. Transfer to large bowl.

4 Add soy sauce mixture to skillet; bring to a boil. Remove from heat. Stir in shrimp and vegetables; toss gently to coat.

PER SERVING:

calories 147, *total fat* 5g, *carbs* 13g, *net carbs* 11g, *dietary fiber* 2g, *protein* 15g

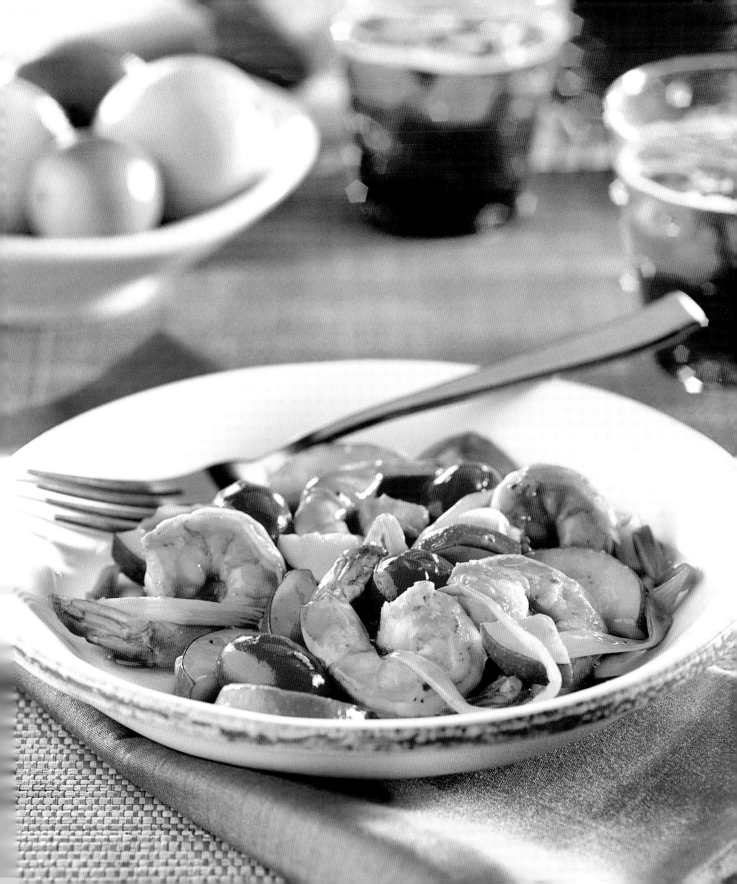

MISO SALMON OVER
GARLICKY SPINACH

makes 4 servings

1½ tablespoons red miso

1 teaspoon minced ginger

¼ teaspoon red pepper flakes

1 tablespoon plus 2 teaspoons water, divided

4 skinless salmon fillets (5 ounces each)

4 cloves garlic, minced

1 bag (10 ounces) fresh spinach leaves or baby spinach

1 Preheat broiler. Combine miso, ginger and red pepper flakes in medium bowl; stir in 2 teaspoons water until blended. Reserve ½ teaspoon mixture in small bowl; spread remaining mixture over top of salmon. Place fish on broiler pan or baking sheet.

2 Broil 4 to 5 inches from heat source 5 to 6 minutes or until fish is opaque in center.

3 Meanwhile, spray large skillet with nonstick cooking spray; heat over medium heat. Add garlic; cook and stir 2 minutes. Stir remaining 1 tablespoon water into reserved miso mixture; mix well. Stir into garlic in skillet. Add spinach to skillet; cook 1 to 2 minutes or just until wilted, turning with tongs constantly. Transfer to serving plates; top with salmon.

NOTE: Miso, which resembles peanut butter, is a paste made from fermented soybeans. It is an essential element of Japanese cooking and comes in many colors and flavors. Miso can be found in Asian and natural foods stores, and in the Asian section of most supermarkets.

PER SERVING:

calories 198, **total fat** 7g, **carbs** 6g, **net carbs** 4g, **dietary fiber** 2g, **protein** 6g

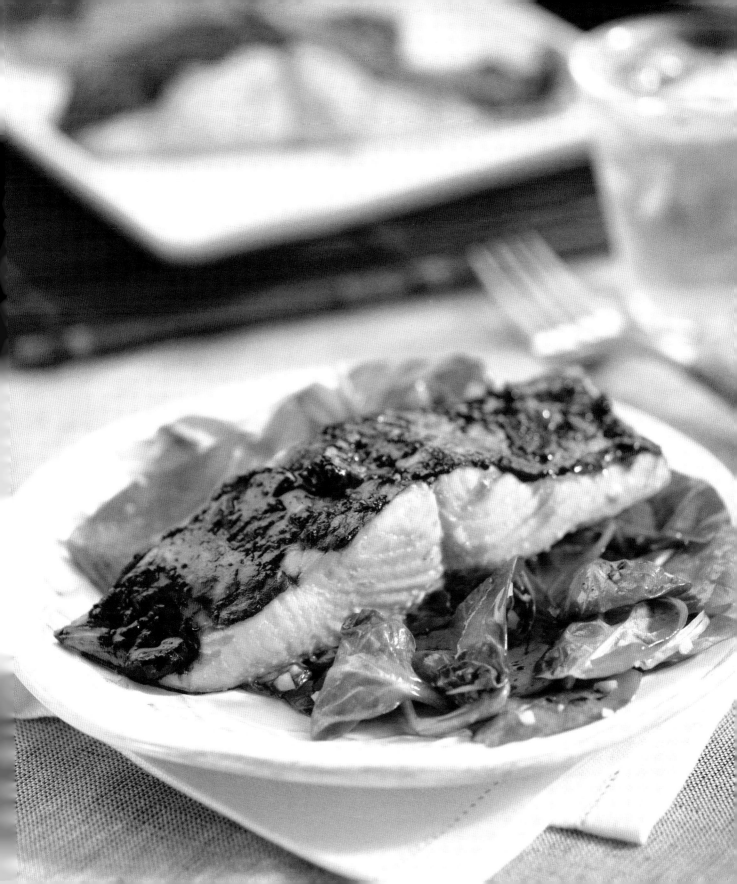

HALIBUT STEAKS WITH TOMATO AND BROCCOLI SAUCE

makes 4 servings

2 tablespoons olive oil

2 cups chopped fresh broccoli

2½ cups diced fresh tomatoes

2 tablespoons lemon juice

1 tablespoon chopped garlic

1 tablespoon chopped fresh tarragon *or* 1 teaspoon dried tarragon

½ teaspoon salt

½ teaspoon black pepper

4 halibut steaks (about 4 ounces each)

Lemon wedges (optional)

1 Heat oil in large skillet over medium heat. Add broccoli; cook and stir 5 minutes. Add tomatoes, lemon juice, garlic, tarragon, salt and pepper; cook and stir 5 minutes.

2 Add halibut; cover and cook 10 minutes or until fish is opaque in center and begins to flake when tested with fork.

3 Divide vegetables evenly among four plates; top with fish. Serve with lemon wedges, if desired.

PER SERVING:

calories 229, *total fat* 10g, *carbs* 10g, *net carbs* 7g, *dietary fiber* 3g, *protein* 26g

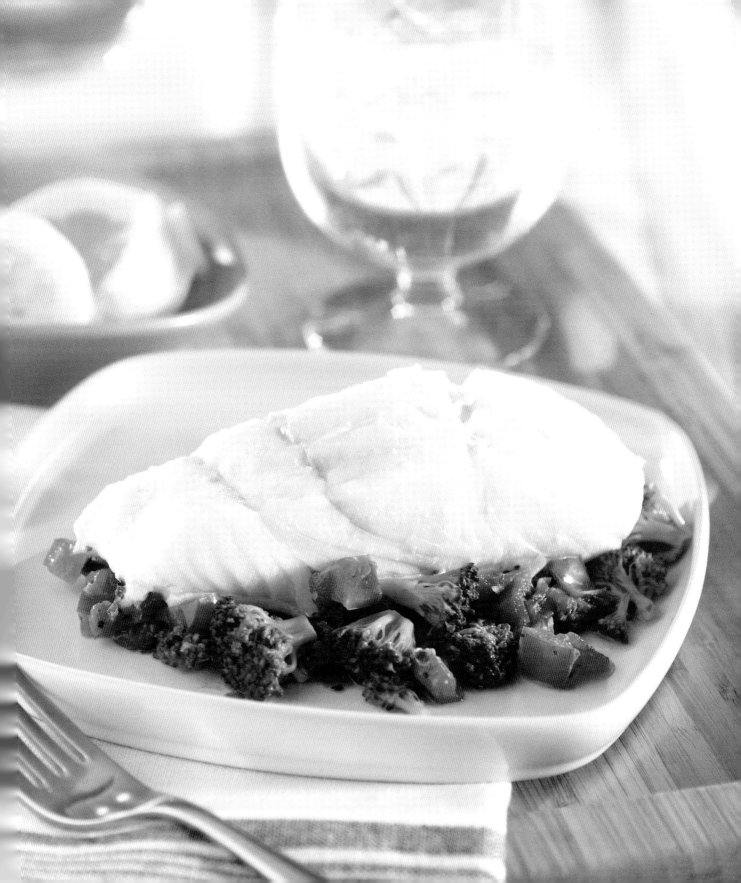

CHIPOTLE SHRIMP
WITH SQUASH RIBBONS

makes 4 servings

2 cloves garlic

1 canned chipotle pepper in adobo sauce, plus 1 teaspoon sauce

2 tablespoons water

2 medium zucchini

2 medium yellow squash

1 teaspoon olive oil

1 small onion, diced

1 medium red bell pepper, cut into strips

8 ounces raw medium shrimp, peeled and deveined

Lime wedges (optional)

1 Combine garlic, chipotle pepper with adobo sauce and water in food processor; process until smooth.

2 Shave squash into ribbons with vegetable peeler, discarding seedy middle of squash.

3 Heat oil in large skillet over high heat. Add onion and bell pepper; cook and stir 1 minute. Add shrimp and chipotle mixture; cook and stir 2 minutes. Add squash; cook and stir 1 to 2 minutes or until shrimp are pink and opaque and squash are heated through and slightly wilted. Serve with lime wedges, if desired.

PER SERVING:

calories 139, *total fat* 3g, *carbs* 13g, *net carbs* 10g, *dietary fiber* 3g, *protein* 14g

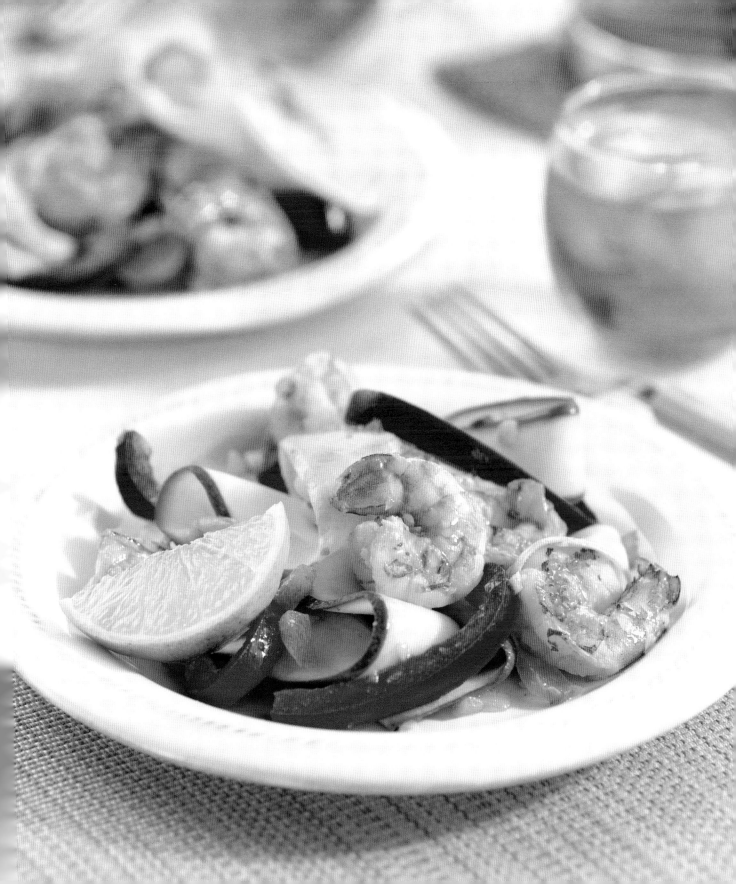

MUSTARD-GRILLED RED SNAPPER

makes 4 servings

½ cup Dijon mustard

1 tablespoon red wine vinegar

1 teaspoon ground red pepper

4 red snapper fillets (about 6 ounces each)

Lemon wedges (optional)

1 Prepare grill for direct cooking. Spray grid with nonstick cooking spray.

2 Combine mustard, vinegar and red pepper in small bowl; mix well. Coat snapper thoroughly with mustard mixture.

3 Grill fish, covered, over medium-high heat 4 minutes per side or until fish begins to flake when tested with fork. Serve with lemon wedges, if desired.

PER SERVING:

calories 210, *total fat* 5g, *carbs* 4g, *net carbs* 3g, *dietary fiber* 1g, *protein* 37g

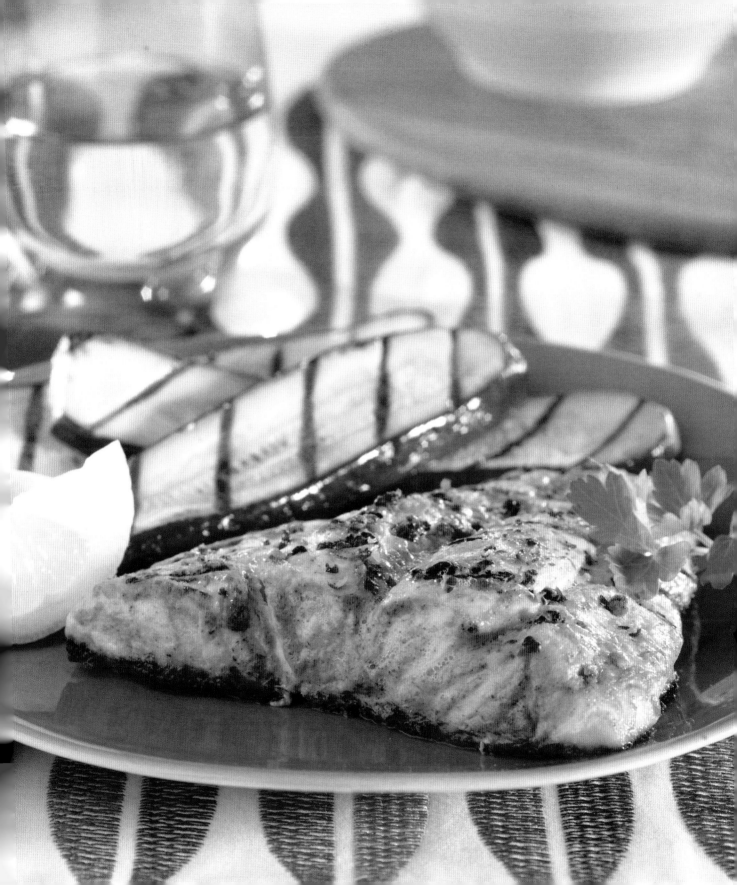

GRILLED SCALLOPS AND VEGETABLES WITH CILANTRO SAUCE

makes 4 servings

1 teaspoon hot chili oil

1 teaspoon dark sesame oil

1 green onion, chopped

1 tablespoon finely chopped fresh ginger

1 cup reduced-sodium chicken broth

1 cup chopped fresh cilantro

1 pound raw or thawed frozen sea scallops

2 medium zucchini, cut into ½-inch slices

2 medium yellow squash, cut into ½-inch slices

1 medium yellow onion, cut into wedges

8 large mushrooms

1 Prepare grill for direct cooking. Spray grid with nonstick cooking spray. If using wooden skewers, soak in water 20 to 25 minutes before using to prevent burning.

2 Heat chili oil and sesame oil in small saucepan over medium-low heat. Add green onion; cook and stir about 15 seconds or just until fragrant. Add ginger; cook and stir 1 minute. Stir in broth; bring to a boil. Cook until liquid is reduced by half; cool slightly. Pour into blender or food processor; add cilantro and blend until smooth. (Or add cilantro to saucepan and use hand-held immersion blender to blend mixture until smooth.)

3 Thread scallops and vegetables onto four 12-inch skewers.

4 Grill over medium-high heat about 8 minutes per side or until scallops turn opaque. Serve warm with cilantro sauce.

PER SERVING:

calories 194, *total fat* 7g, *carbs* 11g, *net carbs* 8g, *dietary fiber* 3g, *protein* 23g

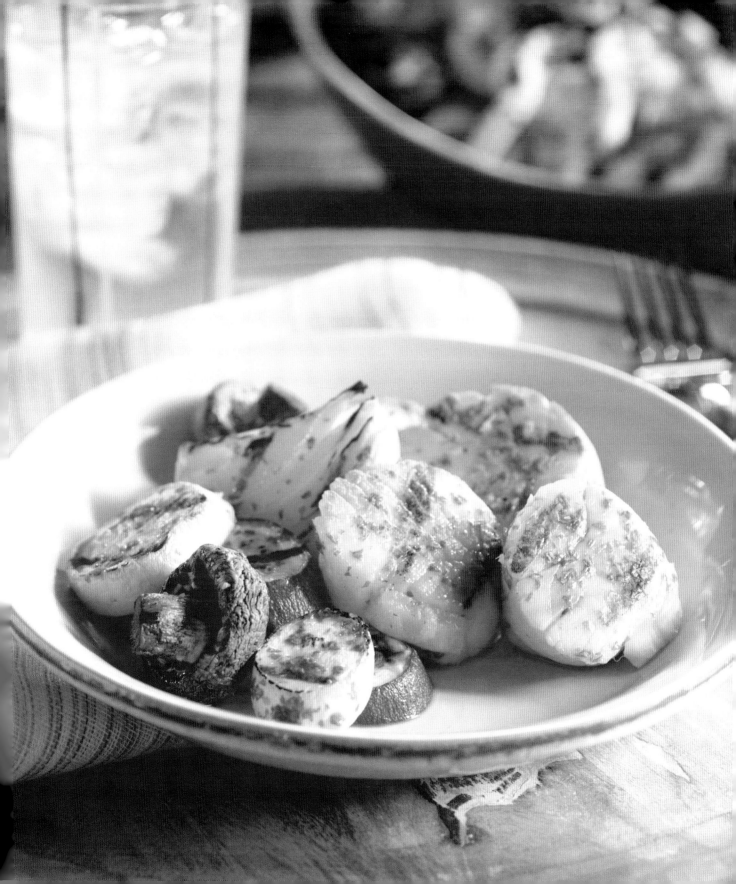

LEMON-GARLIC SALMON WITH TZAZIKI SAUCE

makes 4 servings

- ½ cup diced cucumber
- ¾ teaspoon salt, divided
- 1 cup plain nonfat Greek yogurt
- 2 tablespoons lemon juice, divided
- 1 teaspoon grated lemon peel, divided

- 1 teaspoon minced garlic, divided
- ¼ teaspoon black pepper
- 4 skinless salmon fillets (4 ounces each)

1 Place cucumber in small colander set over small bowl; sprinkle with ¼ teaspoon salt. Drain 1 hour.

2 For sauce, combine yogurt, cucumber, 1 tablespoon lemon juice, ½ teaspoon lemon peel, ½ teaspoon garlic and ¼ teaspoon salt in small bowl; mix well. Cover and refrigerate until ready to use.

3 Combine remaining 1 tablespoon lemon juice, ½ teaspoon lemon peel, ½ teaspoon garlic, ¼ teaspoon salt and pepper in small bowl; mix well. Rub evenly over salmon.

4 Heat nonstick grill pan over medium-high heat. Cook fish 5 minutes per side or until fish begins to flake when tested with fork. Serve with sauce.

PER SERVING:

calories 243, *total fat* 12g, *carbs* 3g, *net carbs* 3g, *dietary fiber* 0g, *protein* 29g

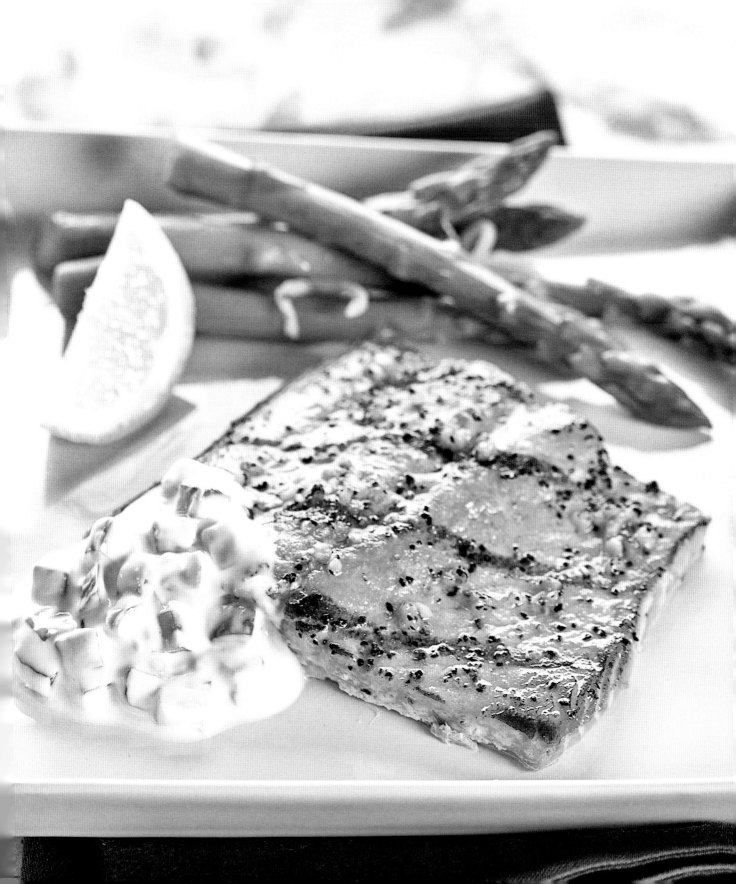

EASY SHRIMP SCAMPI

makes 8 servings

¼ cup (½ stick) plus 2 tablespoons butter

6 to 8 cloves garlic, minced

1½ pounds large raw shrimp (about 16), peeled and deveined (with tails on)

6 green onions, thinly sliced

¼ cup dry white wine or chicken broth

Juice of 1 lemon (about 2 tablespoons)

¼ cup chopped fresh parsley

Salt and black pepper

Lemon slices (optional)

1 To clarify butter, place in small saucepan; heat over low heat until melted. *Do not stir.* Skim off white foam that forms on top. Strain clarified butter through cheesecloth into glass measuring cup to yield ⅓ cup. Discard cheesecloth and milky residue at bottom of pan.

2 Heat clarified butter in large skillet over medium heat. Add garlic; cook and stir 1 to 2 minutes or until softened but not browned.

3 Add shrimp, green onions, wine and lemon juice; cook and stir 3 to 4 minutes or until shrimp are pink and opaque.

4 Stir in parsley; season with salt and pepper. Garnish with lemon slices.

PER SERVING:

calories 150, *total fat* 10g, *carbs* 3g, *net carbs* 3g, *dietary fiber* 0g, *protein* 12g

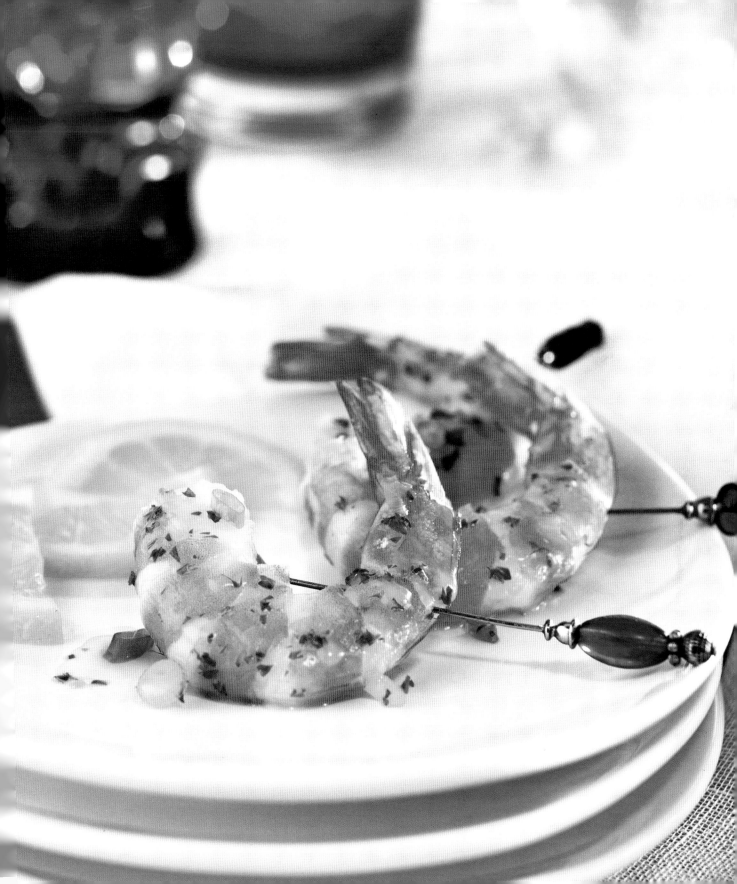

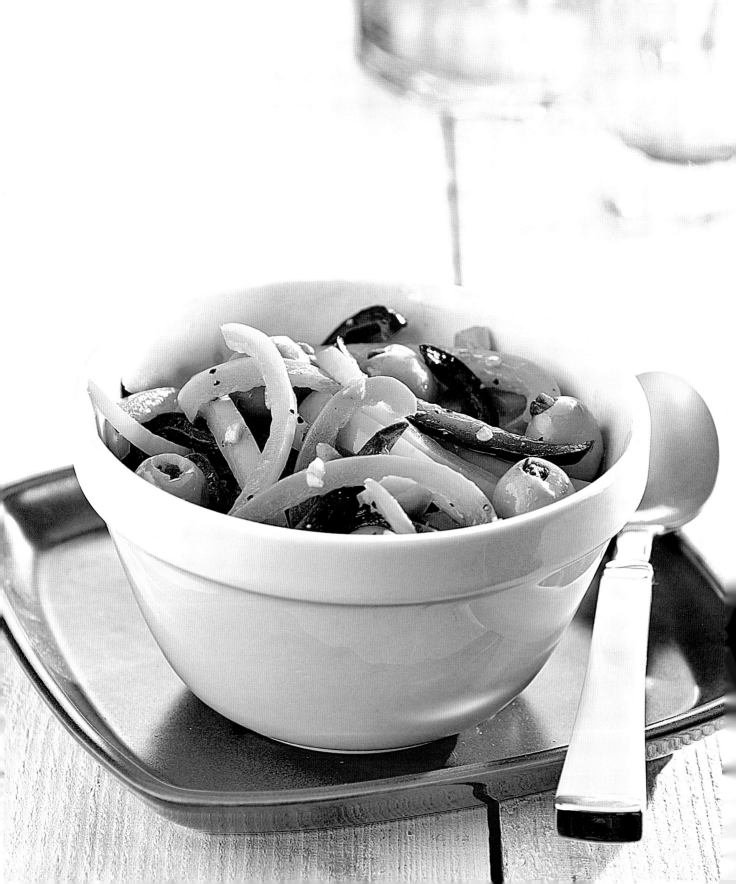

VEGETABLES

PEPERONATA

makes 4 to 5 servings

1 tablespoon extra virgin olive oil

4 large red, yellow and/or orange bell peppers, cut into thin strips

2 cloves garlic, coarsely chopped

12 pimiento-stuffed green olives or pitted black olives, cut into halves

2 to 3 tablespoons white or red wine vinegar

¼ teaspoon salt

¼ teaspoon black pepper

1 Heat oil in large skillet over medium-high heat. Add bell peppers; cook 8 to 9 minutes or until edges begin to brown, stirring frequently.

2 Reduce heat to medium. Add garlic; cook and stir 1 to 2 minutes. *Do not allow garlic to brown.* Add olives, vinegar, salt and black pepper; cook 1 to 2 minutes or until all liquid has evaporated.

NOTE: Peperonata is a very versatile dish. It can be served hot as a condiment or as a side dish with meat dishes. It can also be chilled and served as part of an antipasti selection.

PER SERVING:

calories 89, *total fat* 5g, *carbs* 8g, *net carbs* 5g, *dietary fiber* 3g, *protein* 1g

CREAMY PARMESAN SPINACH

makes 6 servings

2 **tablespoons butter, divided**

1 **cup finely chopped yellow onion**

2 **packages (10 ounces each) fresh spinach, divided**

3 **ounces cream cheese, cut into pieces**

½ **teaspoon garlic powder**

¼ **teaspoon ground nutmeg**

¼ **teaspoon black pepper**

⅛ **teaspoon salt**

2 **tablespoons grated Parmesan, pecorino or Monterey Jack cheese**

1 Melt 1 tablespoon butter in large skillet over medium-high heat. Add onion; cook and stir 4 minutes or until translucent.

2 Add 1 package spinach; cook and stir 2 minutes or just until wilted. Transfer to medium bowl. Repeat with remaining 1 tablespoon butter and spinach.

3 Return reserved spinach to skillet. Add cream cheese, garlic powder, nutmeg, pepper and salt; cook and stir until cream cheese has completely melted.

4 Sprinkle with Parmesan just before serving.

VARIATION: For a thinner consistency, add 2 to 3 tablespoons milk before adding the Parmesan cheese.

PER SERVING:

calories 130, *total fat* 10g, *carbs* 7g, *net carbs* 5g, *dietary fiber* 2g, *protein* 5g

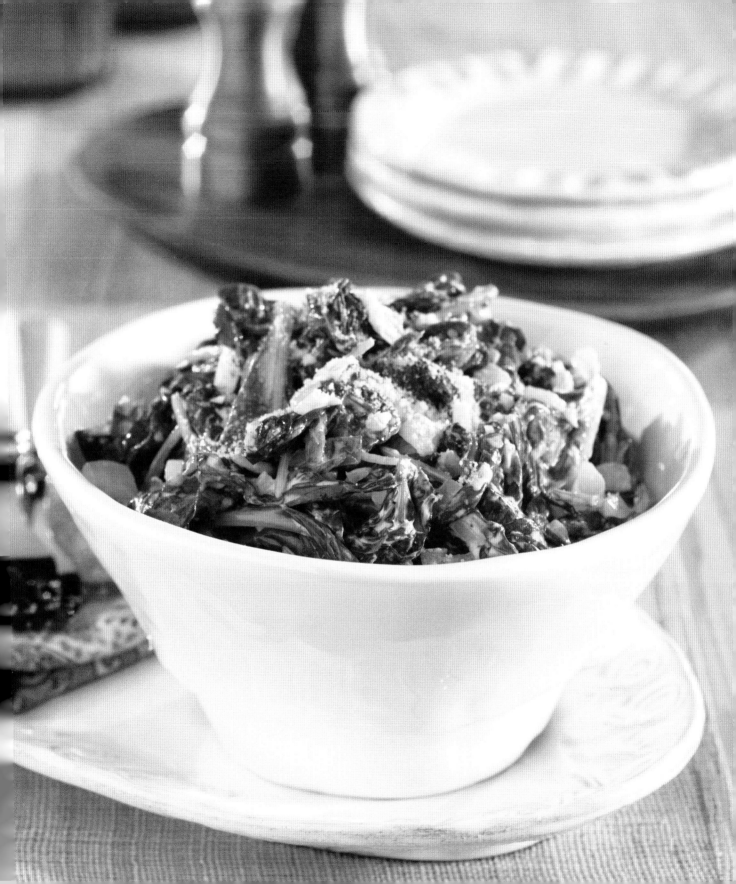

SUMMER SQUASH SKILLET

makes 4 servings

2 **tablespoons butter**

1 **medium sweet or yellow onion, thinly sliced and separated into rings**

2 **medium yellow squash or zucchini** *or* 1 **of each, sliced**

¾ **teaspoon salt**

¼ **teaspoon black pepper**

1 **large tomato, chopped**

¼ **cup chopped fresh basil**

2 **tablespoons grated Parmesan cheese**

1 Melt butter in large skillet over medium-high heat. Add onion; stir to coat with butter. Cover and cook 3 minutes. Uncover; cook and stir over medium heat 3 minutes or until onion is golden brown.

2 Add squash, salt and pepper; cover and cook 5 minutes, stirring once. Add tomato; cook, uncovered, 2 minutes or until squash is tender. Stir in basil; sprinkle with cheese.

PER SERVING:

calories 97, *total fat* 7g, *carbs* 7g, *net carbs* 5g, *dietary fiber* 2g, *protein* 3g

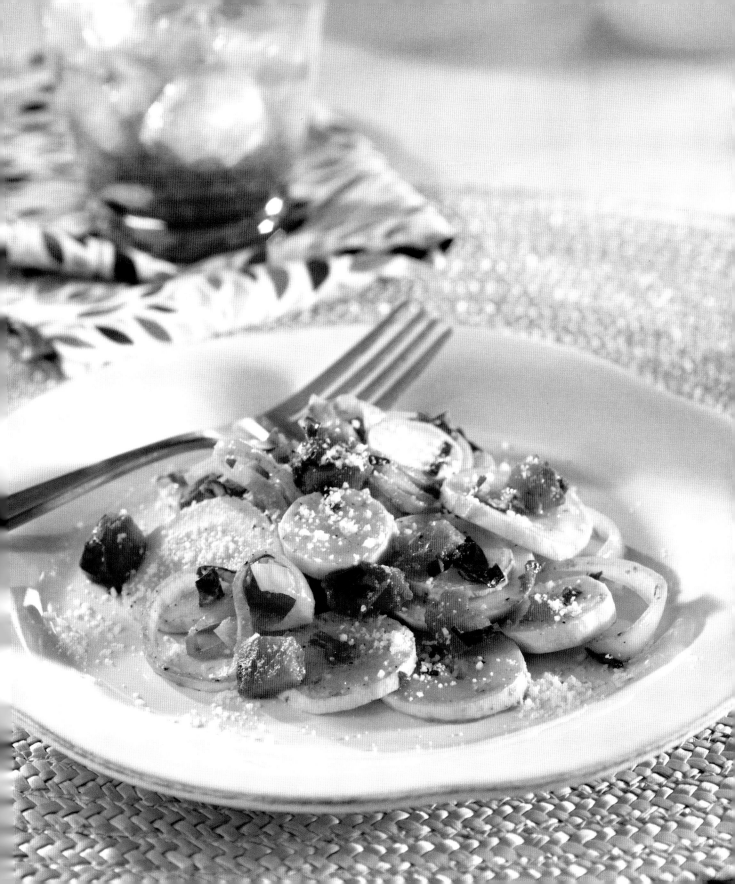

SMOKY KALE CHIFFONADE

makes 4 servings

12 ounces fresh young kale or mustard greens

3 slices bacon

2 tablespoons crumbled blue cheese

1 Rinse kale well in large bowl of water; drain in colander. Discard any discolored leaves; trim away tough stem ends. To prepare chiffonade, roll up leaves jelly-roll style; cut crosswise into ½-inch slices. Separate into strips.

2 Cook bacon in medium skillet over medium heat until crisp. Remove to paper towel-lined plate. Drain all but 1 tablespoon drippings from skillet.

3 Add kale to skillet; cook and stir over medium-high heat 2 to 3 minutes until wilted and tender.*

4 Crumble bacon. Add bacon and blue cheese to kale; toss gently.

If using mustard greens, cook 4 to 6 minutes or until wilted and tender.

NOTE: "Chiffonade" in French literally means "made of rags." In cooking, it means "cut into thin strips."

PER SERVING:

calories 66, *total fat* 4g, *carbs* 5g, *net carbs* 4g, *dietary fiber* 1g, *protein* 4g

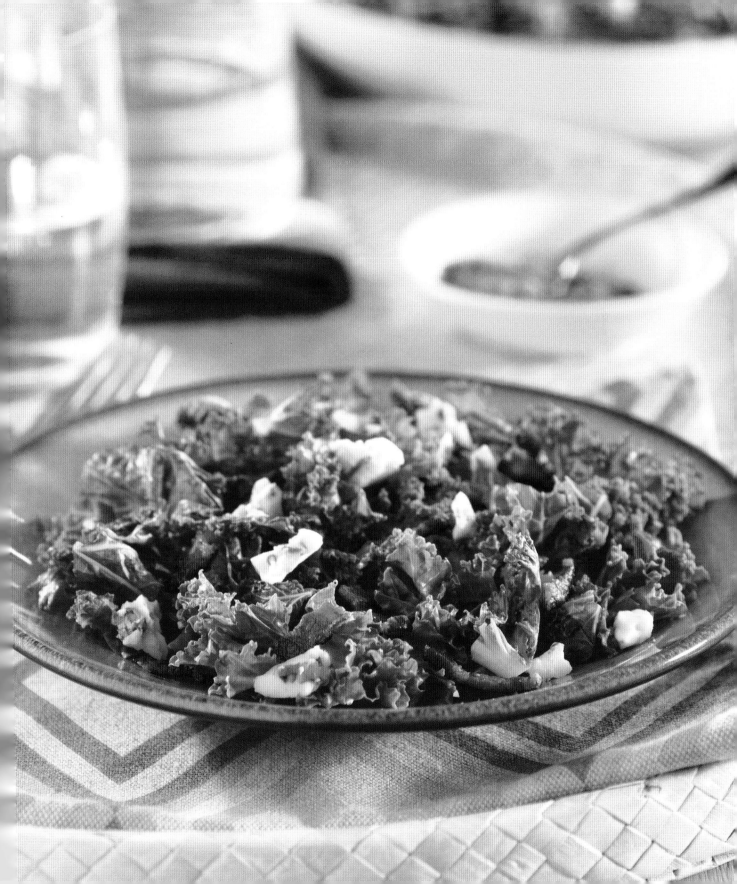

ZOODLES IN TOMATO SAUCE

makes 8 servings

3 teaspoons olive oil, divided

2 cloves garlic

1 tablespoon tomato paste

1 can (28 ounces) whole tomatoes, undrained

1 teaspoon dried oregano

½ teaspoon salt

2 large zucchini (about 16 ounces each), ends trimmed, cut into 3-inch pieces

¼ cup shredded Parmesan cheese

1 Heat 2 teaspoons oil in medium saucepan over medium heat. Add garlic; cook and stir 1 minute or until fragrant but not browned. Add tomato paste; cook and stir 30 seconds. Add tomatoes with juice, oregano and salt; break up tomatoes with wooden spoon. Bring to a simmer. Reduce heat to low; cook 30 minutes or until thickened.

2 Meanwhile, spiral zucchini with fine spiral blade. Heat remaining 1 teaspoon oil in large skillet over medium-high heat. Add zucchini; cook 4 to 5 minutes or until tender, stirring frequently.

3 Transfer zucchini to serving plates; top with tomato sauce and cheese.

TIP: If you don't have a spiralizer, cut the zucchini into ribbons with a mandoline or sharp knife.

PER SERVING:

calories 70, *total fat* 3g, *carbs* 8g, *net carbs* 5g, *dietary fiber* 3g, *protein* 4g

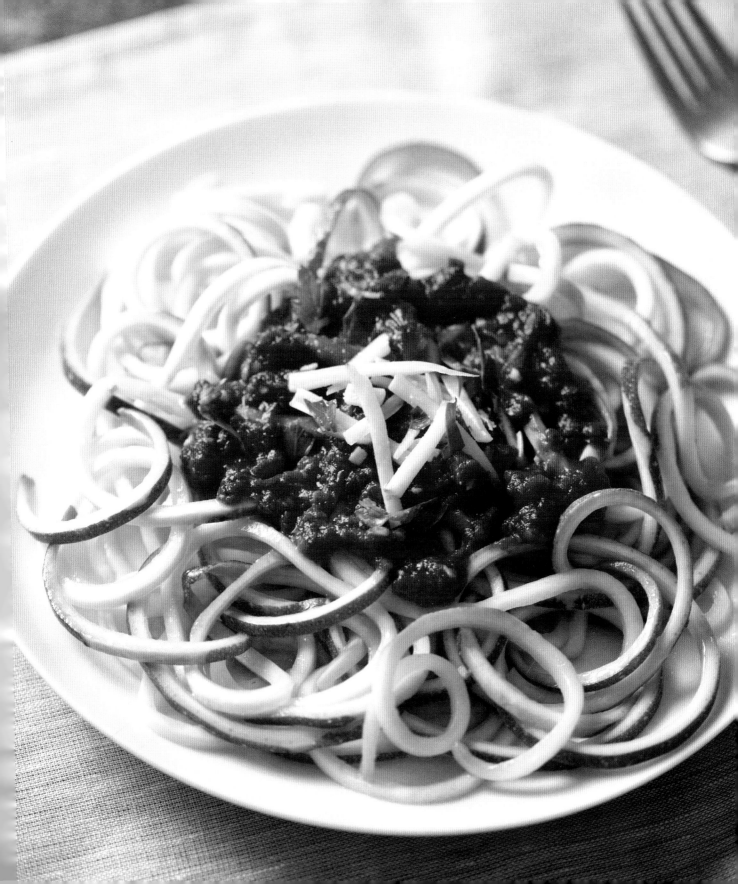

ASPARAGUS WITH CREAMY GARLIC DRESSING

makes 4 servings

2 tablespoons sour cream

1 tablespoon buttermilk or whipping cream

1 teaspoon grated lemon peel, plus additional for garnish

1 clove garlic, minced

Salt and black pepper

24 asparagus spears, trimmed and diagonally cut into 1-inch pieces

1 Whisk sour cream, buttermilk, 1 teaspoon lemon peel and garlic in small bowl until well blended. Season with salt and pepper.

2 Place asparagus in large skillet; add just enough water to just cover. Season with salt and bring to a boil over high heat. Reduce heat to a simmer; cook 3 to 5 minutes or until asparagus is crisp-tender. Drain asparagus; rinse under cold water to stop cooking.

3 Place asparagus in serving bowl. Add dressing; stir gently to coat. Garnish with additional lemon peel.

PER SERVING:

calories 34, *total fat* 0g, *carbs* 7g, *net carbs* 4g, *dietary fiber* 3g, *protein* 3g

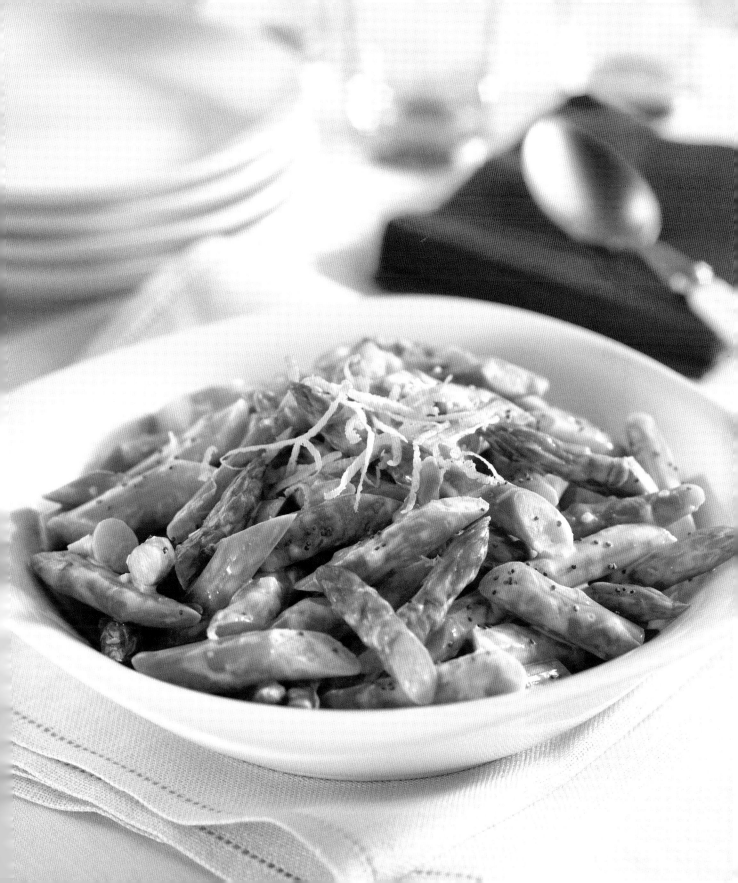

SZECHUAN GRILLED MUSHROOMS

makes 4 servings

1 pound large mushrooms

2 tablespoons soy sauce

2 teaspoons peanut oil

1 teaspoon dark sesame oil

1 clove garlic, minced

½ teaspoon crushed Szechuan peppercorns or red pepper flakes

1 Place mushrooms in large resealable food storage bag. Combine soy sauce, peanut oil, sesame oil, garlic and Szechuan peppercorns in small bowl; mix well. Pour over mushrooms. Seal bag; turn to coat. Marinate at room temperature 15 minutes.

2 Prepare grill for direct cooking. If using wooden skewers, soak in water 20 to 25 minutes before using to prevent burning. Thread mushrooms onto skewers.

3 Grill or broil mushrooms 5 inches from heat 10 minutes or until lightly browned, turning once. Serve immediately.

PER SERVING:

calories 61, *total fat* 4g, *carbs* 5g, *net carbs* 3g, *dietary fiber* 2g, *protein* 4g

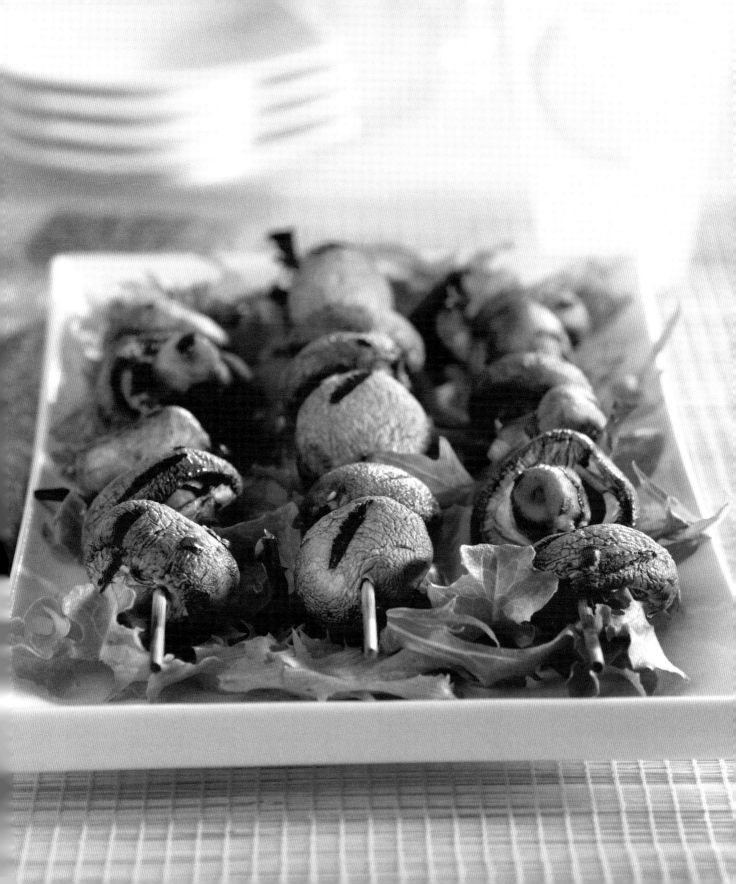

BROCCOLI ITALIAN STYLE

makes 4 servings

1¼ pounds fresh broccoli

2 tablespoons lemon juice

1 teaspoon extra virgin olive oil

1 clove garlic, minced

1 teaspoon chopped fresh Italian parsley

Dash black pepper

1 Trim broccoli, discarding tough stems. Cut broccoli into florets with 2-inch stems. Peel remaining stems; cut into ½-inch slices.

2 Bring 1 quart water to a boil in large saucepan over medium-high heat. Add broccoli; return to a boil. Cook 3 to 5 minutes or until broccoli is tender. Drain well; transfer to serving dish.

3 Whisk lemon juice, oil, garlic, parsley and pepper in small bowl until well blended. Pour over broccoli; toss to coat. Cover and let stand 1 hour before serving to allow flavors to blend. Serve at room temperature.

PER SERVING:

calories 44, *total fat* 2g, *carbs* 7g, *net carbs* 4g, *dietary fiber* 3g, *protein* 3g

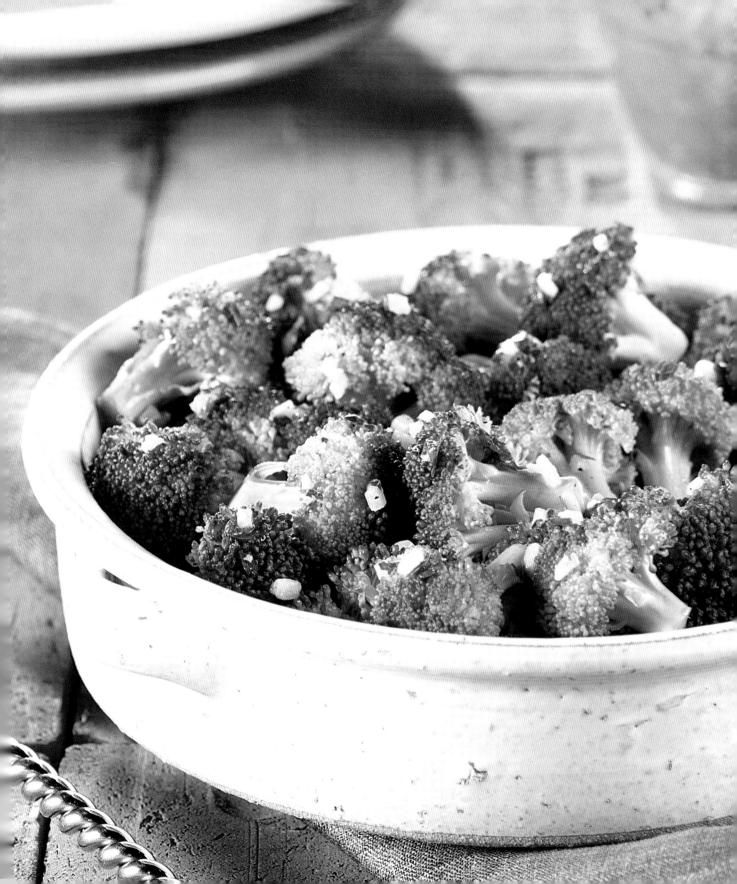

ZUCCHINI FETA CASSEROLE

makes 4 servings

4 medium zucchini	2 tablespoons chopped fresh parsley
1 tablespoon butter	2 teaspoons chopped fresh marjoram
2 eggs, beaten	Dash hot pepper sauce
½ cup grated Parmesan cheese	Salt and black pepper
⅓ cup crumbled feta cheese	

1 Preheat oven to 375°F. Spray 2-quart casserole with nonstick cooking spray.

2 Grate zucchini; drain in colander. Melt butter in large skillet over medium heat. Add zucchini; cook and stir until slightly browned.

3 Remove from heat; stir in eggs, Parmesan, feta, parsley, marjoram, hot pepper sauce, salt and black pepper until well blended. Pour into prepared casserole.

4 Bake 35 minutes or until hot and bubbly.

PER SERVING:

calories 220, *total fat* 14g, *carbs* 12g, *net carbs* 9g, *dietary fiber* 3g, *protein* 15g

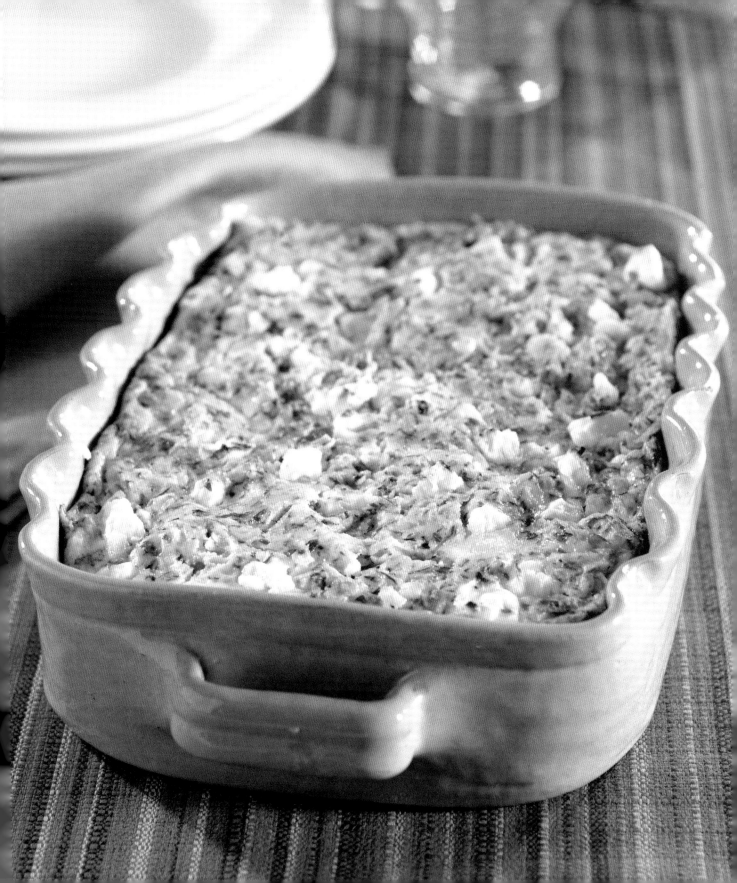

SAUTÉED KALE WITH MUSHROOMS AND BACON

makes 4 servings

1 slice bacon, chopped

½ cup sliced shallots

1 package (4 ounces) sliced mixed exotic mushrooms *or* 2 cups sliced button mushrooms

10 cups (8 ounces) loosely packed torn fresh kale leaves (no tough stems)*

2 tablespoons water

½ teaspoon black pepper

Look for 16-ounce bags of ready-to-cook fresh kale leaves in the produce section of the supermarket.

1 Cook bacon in large skillet over medium heat 5 minutes. Add shallots; cook and stir 3 minutes. Add mushrooms; cook 8 minutes, stirring occasionally.

2 Add kale and water; cover and cook 5 minutes. Uncover; cook and stir 5 minutes or until kale is crisp-tender, stirring occasionally. Season with pepper.

PER SERVING:

calories 90, *total fat* 4g, *carbs* 11g, *net carbs* 8g, *dietary fiber* 3g, *protein* 4g

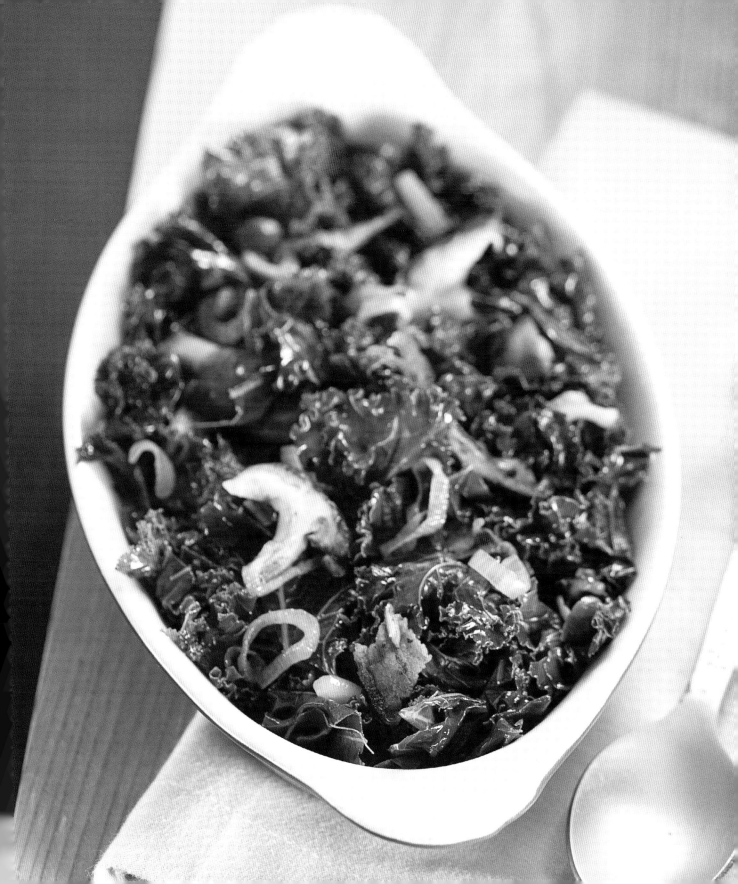

METRIC CONVERSION CHART

VOLUME MEASUREMENTS (dry)

1/8 teaspoon = 0.5 mL
1/4 teaspoon = 1 mL
1/2 teaspoon = 2 mL
3/4 teaspoon = 4 mL
1 teaspoon = 5 mL
1 tablespoon = 15 mL
2 tablespoons = 30 mL
1/4 cup = 60 mL
1/3 cup = 75 mL
1/2 cup = 125 mL
2/3 cup = 150 mL
3/4 cup = 175 mL
1 cup = 250 mL
2 cups = 1 pint = 500 mL
3 cups = 750 mL
4 cups = 1 quart = 1 L

VOLUME MEASUREMENTS (fluid)

1 fluid ounce (2 tablespoons) = 30 mL
4 fluid ounces (1/2 cup) = 125 mL
8 fluid ounces (1 cup) = 250 mL
12 fluid ounces (1 1/2 cups) = 375 mL
16 fluid ounces (2 cups) = 500 mL

WEIGHTS (mass)

1/2 ounce = 15 g
1 ounce = 30 g
3 ounces = 90 g
4 ounces = 120 g
8 ounces = 225 g
10 ounces = 285 g
12 ounces = 360 g
16 ounces = 1 pound = 450 g

DIMENSIONS

1/16 inch = 2 mm
1/8 inch = 3 mm
1/4 inch = 6 mm
1/2 inch = 1.5 cm
3/4 inch = 2 cm
1 inch = 2.5 cm

OVEN TEMPERATURES

250°F = 120°C
275°F = 140°C
300°F = 150°C
325°F = 160°C
350°F = 180°C
375°F = 190°C
400°F = 200°C
425°F = 220°C
450°F = 230°C

BAKING PAN SIZES

Utensil	Size in Inches/Quarts	Metric Volume	Size in Centimeters
Baking or Cake Pan (square or rectangular)	8×8×2	2 L	20×20×5
	9×9×2	2.5 L	23×23×5
	12×8×2	3 L	30×20×5
	13×9×2	3.5 L	33×23×5
Loaf Pan	8×4×3	1.5 L	20×10×7
	9×5×3	2 L	23×13×7
Round Layer Cake Pan	8×1½	1.2 L	20×4
	9×1½	1.5 L	23×4
Pie Plate	8×1¼	750 mL	20×3
	9×1¼	1 L	23×3
Baking Dish or Casserole	1 quart	1 L	—
	1½ quart	1.5 L	—
	2 quart	2 L	—